TABLE OF CONTENTS

DINNER RECIPES--------------------------------------121

CONCLUSION -----------------------------------192

INTRODUCTION

In an era marked by the incessant quest for optimal health and sustainable weight management, the DASH (Dietary Approaches to Stop Hypertension) diet stands as a beacon of nutritional wisdom. Originally crafted to combat hypertension, this dietary approach has transcended its primary purpose, evolving into a holistic lifestyle strategy that not only cultivates heart health but also champions weight loss and overall well-being.

The DASH diet is far more than a fleeting dietary trend; it's a well-founded nutritional framework meticulously crafted by experts in health and nutrition. It revolves around a harmonious integration of whole foods, emphasizing the consumption of fruits, vegetables, lean proteins, whole grains, and low-fat dairy products while curbing the intake of sodium, sugary treats, and processed foods.

At its core, the DASH diet isn't just about slashing sodium intake to tame blood pressure; it's a holistic and sustainable dietary regimen that extends its benefits beyond cardiovascular health. By fortifying the body with an abundance of nutrient-dense, low-calorie foods, the DASH diet becomes an invaluable ally in the pursuit of weight loss and optimal physical wellness.

DASH diet isn't restrictive; rather, it's liberating in its emphasis on diverse, nutrient-dense foods. By promoting the consumption of wholesome, unprocessed foods rich in vitamins, minerals, and fiber, it naturally aids in weight management while nourishing the body. Unlike fad diets that promise rapid weight loss at the expense of sustainability, the DASH diet is a sustainable, long-term solution. Its emphasis on balanced meals and portion control cultivates habits that can be maintained for life.

Supported by scientific research, the DASH diet's effectiveness in reducing weight, enhancing metabolic health, and improving overall wellness is well-documented. It's a proven approach endorsed by health professionals worldwide.

Gone are the days of crash diets that leave you famished and fatigued. With the DASH diet, it's about sustainable change. It's about crafting a way of eating that not only trims waistlines but also nurtures overall health. It's a testament to the idea that weight loss need not be a grueling journey but rather a fulfilling exploration of delicious, nourishing foods.

Throughout this guide, you'll delve deep into the intricate tapestry of the DASH diet. We'll unravel the science behind its effectiveness, decode its fundamental principles, and arm you with the tools to embark on a transformative journey.

From understanding the nutritional alchemy behind DASH-approved foods to crafting delectable meals that tantalize taste buds while shedding inches, this guide is your compass in navigating the realm of healthy weight loss through the DASH diet.

Prepare to delve into a world of nourishment, discover culinary delights, and embrace a lifestyle that not only transforms your body but elevates your entire well-being. Welcome to the transformative realm of the DASH diet—a path to weight loss and vibrant health!

CHAPTER ONE

WHAT IS DASH DIET?

The DASH diet, which stands for Dietary Approaches to Stop Hypertension, is an eating plan primarily designed to help lower blood pressure and reduce the risk of hypertension (high blood pressure). Developed by the National Heart, Lung, and Blood Institute (NHLBI), it's a flexible and balanced eating plan that focuses on promoting heart health and overall well-being.

Significance for Weight Loss:

The DASH diet's significance for weight loss lies in its focus on whole, nutrient-dense foods and its ability to provide a balanced approach to eating. By emphasizing a variety of foods that are low in calories but high in nutrients, it supports weight loss while still ensuring adequate nutrition.

Additionally, the DASH diet doesn't involve severe restrictions or deprivation, making it a sustainable approach for those aiming to lose weight. Its emphasis on portion control, whole foods, and a balanced intake of nutrients contributes to its effectiveness in not only managing blood pressure but also aiding in weight management.

Ultimately, the DASH diet serves as a versatile and adaptable eating plan that promotes overall health, encourages healthy eating habits, and can be tailored to individual needs and preferences.

THE PRIMARY PURPOSE OF THE DASH DIET

The primary purpose of the DASH (Dietary Approaches to Stop Hypertension) diet is to prevent and manage hypertension, commonly known as high blood pressure. However, the diet's benefits extend beyond blood pressure control and are also effective for overall heart health and reducing the risk of other chronic diseases.

Here are the detailed aspects of the primary purpose of the DASH diet:

1. Lowering Blood Pressure:

Emphasis on Nutrient-Rich Foods: The DASH diet encourages the consumption of fruits, vegetables, whole grains, lean proteins, and low-fat dairy products. These foods are rich in potassium, magnesium, calcium, and fiber, which have been shown to help lower blood pressure.

Reducing Sodium Intake: The diet emphasizes limiting sodium intake to lower blood pressure. By focusing on whole, unprocessed foods and reducing high-sodium processed foods, it helps maintain healthier blood pressure levels.

2. Cardiovascular Health:

Reducing Risk Factors: The DASH diet aids in reducing several risk factors associated with heart disease, such as high blood pressure, high cholesterol levels, and high triglycerides.

Promotion of Healthy Fats: While the DASH diet limits saturated and trans fats, it encourages the consumption of healthy fats found in sources like nuts, seeds, and certain oils, which can contribute to better heart health.

3. Weight Management:

Focus on Nutrient-Dense Foods: The DASH diet emphasizes nutrient-dense foods that are lower in calories, helping individuals maintain a healthy weight or lose weight if needed.

Balanced Approach: By promoting a balanced intake of whole foods, lean proteins, and complex carbohydrates, the diet supports weight loss without extreme restrictions, making it easier to sustain in the long term.

4. Overall Health and Disease Prevention:

Rich in Nutrients: The DASH diet includes foods that are abundant in vitamins, minerals, and antioxidants, providing a wide array of nutrients that support overall health and may help reduce the risk of chronic diseases like diabetes, certain cancers, and osteoporosis.

Lifestyle and Dietary Balance: The diet isn't just about food choices; it encourages a comprehensive approach to a healthier lifestyle, combining nutrition with physical activity and stress management.

The DASH diet's primary goal of managing blood pressure serves as a cornerstone for overall health and well-being. By promoting a diet rich in essential nutrients, balanced macronutrients, and a reduction in sodium intake, it not only helps manage hypertension but also significantly contributes to improving cardiovascular health, maintaining a healthy weight, and reducing the risk of chronic diseases. Its focus on a sustainable and balanced approach makes it a valuable dietary pattern for promoting lifelong health and wellness.

THE PRINCIPLES BEHIND THE DIET

The DASH (Dietary Approaches to Stop Hypertension) diet is based on several principles that guide its approach to promoting heart health, managing blood pressure, and supporting overall well-being. These principles revolve around dietary patterns that emphasize specific food groups, nutrient intake, and overall lifestyle changes. Here are the key principles behind the DASH diet:

1. Emphasis on Fruits and Vegetables:

Abundant Consumption: Encourages consuming a variety of fruits and vegetables daily. These foods are rich in vitamins, minerals, antioxidants, and fiber, promoting heart health and overall well-being.

Colorful Variety: Recommends a diverse range of colorful fruits and vegetables to ensure a broad spectrum of nutrients.

2. Inclusion of Whole Grains:

Preference for Whole Grains: Emphasizes whole grains over refined grains. Whole grains like brown rice, quinoa, whole wheat bread, and oats offer more fiber, vitamins, and minerals, contributing to heart health and better blood pressure management.

3. Lean Protein Sources:

Lean Protein Choices: Encourages lean sources of protein such as poultry, fish, beans, lentils, nuts, and seeds. These are lower in saturated fats and provide essential amino acids without contributing to elevated cholesterol levels.

4. Low-Fat Dairy:

Moderation in Fat Intake: Recommends low-fat or fat-free dairy products like milk, yogurt, and cheese to reduce saturated fat intake while still providing essential nutrients like calcium and vitamin D.

5. Reduction in Sodium Intake:

Limiting Sodium: Advocates for reducing sodium intake by choosing fresh foods over processed and packaged options. This helps manage blood pressure levels and reduces the risk of hypertension.

6. Moderate Consumption of Sweets and Sugary Beverages:

Moderation in Added Sugars: Encourages limiting the intake of sweets, sugary beverages, and foods high in added sugars to control calorie intake and prevent excessive sugar consumption.

7. Portion Control and Balanced Eating:

Portion Awareness: Promotes portion control and mindful eating to maintain a healthy calorie balance.

Balanced Macronutrients: Encourages a balanced intake of carbohydrates, proteins, and healthy fats to support overall health and energy levels.

8. Physical Activity and Lifestyle Changes:

Integration of Exercise: While not exclusively a dietary principle, the DASH diet advocates incorporating regular physical activity for optimal health and weight management.

Stress Management: Recognizes the importance of stress reduction and relaxation techniques for overall health and well-being.

The principles of the DASH diet emphasize a holistic approach to nutrition and lifestyle. By focusing on nutrient-rich foods, moderation in certain food groups, and lifestyle changes like exercise and stress management, the diet aims to support heart health, manage blood pressure, promote weight loss, and reduce the risk of chronic diseases. Its principles encourage a sustainable and balanced approach to eating that can be adopted for long-term health benefits.

HOW THE DASH DIET PROMOTE OVERALL HEALTH

The DASH (Dietary Approaches to Stop Hypertension) diet is renowned not only for its efficacy in managing blood pressure but also for its ability to promote overall health and well-being. Its core principles and nutritional components contribute to various aspects of health beyond just cardiovascular benefits. Here's how the DASH diet promotes overall health:

1. Heart Health and Blood Pressure Management:

Reducing Hypertension: The primary aim of the DASH diet is to lower high blood pressure. By emphasizing nutrient-dense foods and limiting sodium intake, it helps manage hypertension, reducing the risk of heart disease, stroke, and other cardiovascular conditions.

2. Nutrient-Rich Foods:

Abundance of Nutrients: The diet encourages the consumption of fruits, vegetables, whole grains, lean proteins, and low-fat dairy, which are rich in vitamins, minerals, antioxidants, and fiber.

Supports Immune Function: Nutrient-dense foods support a strong immune system, helping the body fight off illnesses and infections.

3. Weight Management and Metabolic Health:

Balanced Macronutrients: Emphasizing a balance of carbohydrates, proteins, and healthy fats aids in weight management and supports a healthy metabolism.

Reduced Risk of Obesity: The focus on whole, low-calorie, and filling foods can contribute to weight loss or maintenance, reducing the risk of obesity-related conditions.

4. Reduced Risk of Chronic Diseases:

Preventing Diabetes: The DASH diet's emphasis on whole grains, fruits, and vegetables and its ability to help manage weight may lower the risk of type 2 diabetes.

Lower Risk of Certain Cancers: The diet's high-fiber content from fruits, vegetables, and whole grains may help reduce the risk of certain cancers.

5. Improved Digestive Health:

High Fiber Content: The diet's emphasis on fiber-rich foods supports digestive health, prevents constipation, and fosters a healthy gut microbiome.

6. Better Cholesterol Levels:

Healthy Fats: While limiting saturated fats, the diet promotes sources of healthy fats like nuts, seeds, and certain oils, which can improve cholesterol levels and support heart health.

7. Lifestyle Integration:

Physical Activity: Though not strictly dietary, the DASH diet often integrates recommendations for regular physical activity, which is crucial for overall health and weight management.

Stress Reduction: Encouraging stress management techniques complements the diet's holistic approach to health.

The DASH diet's multifaceted approach to nutrition, focusing on nutrient-rich foods, portion control, and lifestyle modifications, extends well beyond blood pressure management. By promoting heart health, weight management, reduced risk of chronic diseases, and overall well-being, the DASH diet stands as a comprehensive dietary approach that fosters holistic health. Its principles advocate a balanced and sustainable lifestyle that supports long-term health benefits for individuals of all ages.

THE BENEFITS OF THE DASH DIET FOR WEIGHT LOSS.

The DASH (Dietary Approaches to Stop Hypertension) diet, primarily designed to lower blood pressure, also offers significant benefits for weight loss. Here are the key benefits of the DASH diet in supporting weight loss:

1. Emphasis on Nutrient-Dense Foods:

Low-Calorie, High-Nutrient Content: Encourages the consumption of fruits, vegetables, whole grains, lean proteins, and low-fat dairy, which are nutrient-dense but lower in calories. These foods help in weight management by providing essential nutrients without excessive calories.

2. Portion Control and Balanced Eating:

Promotes Portion Awareness: Emphasizes portion control without strict calorie counting, helping individuals manage their food intake and prevent overeating.

Balanced Macronutrients: Advocates for a balanced intake of carbohydrates, proteins, and healthy fats, supporting satiety and reducing the likelihood of nutrient deficiencies.

3. Supports a Healthy Metabolism:

Balanced Diet Composition: Incorporates a combination of macronutrients that can support a healthy metabolism, aiding in weight loss or maintenance.

4. Lowers Saturated Fat and Added Sugars:

Reduction in Unhealthy Fats: Encourages the limitation of saturated fats and emphasizes healthy fats from sources like nuts and seeds.

Moderation in Sugary Foods: Recommends moderation in added sugars, which can help reduce overall calorie intake and prevent spikes in blood sugar levels.

5. Encourages Whole Foods Over Processed Foods:

Preference for Whole, Unprocessed Foods: Recommends choosing whole, natural foods over highly processed options, which are often higher in calories, unhealthy fats, and added sugars.

6. Sustainable and Balanced Approach:

Not a Fad Diet: The DASH diet is a sustainable and balanced eating plan, promoting lifelong healthy eating habits rather than short-term, restrictive diets.

7. Lifestyle Integration:

Promotes Physical Activity: While not exclusively dietary, the DASH diet often integrates recommendations for regular physical activity, which complements weight loss efforts.

Stress Management: Encourages stress reduction techniques, which can support weight loss by preventing emotional eating and promoting healthier habits.

The DASH diet's focus on whole, nutrient-dense foods, portion control, and balanced macronutrients makes it an effective approach for weight loss. By encouraging healthier food choices, promoting satiety, and supporting a lifestyle conducive to weight management, the DASH diet stands as a sustainable dietary plan that not only aids in lowering blood pressure but also facilitates successful weight loss and maintenance.

The DASH (Dietary Approaches to Stop Hypertension) diet emphasizes specific food groups that are integral to promoting heart health, managing blood pressure, and supporting overall well-being. Here's a breakdown of the food groups recommended in the DASH diet:

1. Fruits:

Variety: Encourages a diverse selection of fruits, including berries, citrus fruits, apples, bananas, melons, and more.

Benefits: Fruits are rich in vitamins, minerals, antioxidants, and fiber, providing essential nutrients while being relatively low in calories.

2. Vegetables:

Colorful Variety: Advocates for consuming a colorful array of vegetables, such as leafy greens, tomatoes, carrots, bell peppers, broccoli, and others.

Nutrient Density: Vegetables are packed with vitamins, minerals, antioxidants, and fiber, contributing to heart health and overall well-being.

3. Whole Grains:

Preference for Whole Grains: Recommends whole grains like brown rice, quinoa, whole wheat bread, oats, barley, and whole grain pasta over refined grains.

Nutrient-Rich: Whole grains are rich in fiber, vitamins, minerals, and antioxidants, offering more nutrients than refined grains.

4. Lean Proteins:

Poultry and Fish: Encourages the consumption of lean protein sources such as chicken, turkey, and fish like salmon, trout, and tuna.

Plant-Based Proteins: Includes beans, lentils, nuts, and seeds as sources of protein, offering plant-based alternatives with lower saturated fat content.

5. Low-Fat Dairy:

Low-Fat or Fat-Free Options: Recommends low-fat or fat-free dairy products like milk, yogurt, and cheese to reduce saturated fat intake.

Calcium and Vitamin D: Provides essential nutrients like calcium and vitamin D for bone health without excessive saturated fats.

6. Nuts, Seeds, and Legumes:

Healthy Fats and Plant-Based Proteins: Encourages the consumption of nuts, seeds, and legumes as sources of healthy fats, fiber, and plant-based proteins.

Walnuts, Almonds, Flaxseeds, Beans, and Lentils: These foods offer a variety of nutrients, including omega-3 fatty acids, fiber, vitamins, and minerals.

7. Fats and Oils:

Healthy Fats: Recommends healthy fats from sources like olive oil, canola oil, avocados, and nuts while limiting saturated and trans fats.

8. Sweets and Added Sugars:

Moderation: Advises moderation in the consumption of sweets, sugary beverages, and foods high in added sugars to control overall calorie intake.

The DASH diet emphasizes a balanced intake of nutrient-rich foods from various food groups, focusing on fruits, vegetables, whole grains, lean proteins, low-fat dairy, nuts, seeds, and legumes. This diverse selection of foods ensures a wide range of essential nutrients while promoting heart health, managing blood pressure, and supporting overall health and well-being.

HOW THESE FOOD GROUPS CONTRIBUTE TO WEIGHT LOSS.

The food groups recommended in the DASH (Dietary Approaches to Stop Hypertension) diet play a crucial role in supporting weight loss due to their nutrient density, fiber content, and overall impact on satiety. Here's how each food group contributes to weight loss within the framework of the DASH diet:

1. Fruits and Vegetables:

Low-Calorie, High-Fiber Content: Fruits and vegetables are low in calories while being rich in fiber, aiding in satiety and reducing overall calorie intake. They also provide essential vitamins, minerals, and antioxidants.

2. Whole Grains:

High in Fiber: Whole grains like brown rice, quinoa, and oats contain more fiber than refined grains, promoting feelings of fullness and reducing the likelihood of overeating.

Sustained Energy: The complex carbohydrates in whole grains provide sustained energy, preventing spikes in blood sugar levels that can lead to cravings.

3. Lean Proteins:

Satiety: Lean protein sources such as poultry, fish, beans, and lentils contribute to feeling full and satisfied after meals, reducing the desire to snack excessively between meals.

Muscle Preservation: Adequate protein intake supports muscle preservation during weight loss, aiding in maintaining a healthy metabolism.

4. Low-Fat Dairy:

Calcium and Protein: Low-fat dairy products offer calcium and protein for bone health and muscle maintenance. Protein also aids in satiety and muscle recovery after exercise.

5. Nuts, Seeds, and Legumes:

Healthy Fats and Protein: Nuts, seeds, and legumes are rich in healthy fats, protein, and fiber, contributing to feelings of fullness and providing essential nutrients without excessive calories.

6. Healthy Fats and Oils:

Satiety: Healthy fats from sources like olive oil and avocados can enhance satiety, helping to control hunger and reduce overall calorie consumption when consumed in moderation.

7. Moderation in Sweets and Added Sugars:

Calorie Control: Limiting sweets and added sugars helps control overall calorie intake, preventing excessive consumption of empty calories that may lead to weight gain.

The food groups recommended in the DASH diet contribute to weight loss by providing a variety of nutrient-dense, low-calorie options that promote feelings of fullness, control hunger, and support overall health. Their high fiber content, balanced macronutrients, and ability to satisfy appetite help individuals manage their weight effectively while ensuring they receive essential nutrients for optimal health.

THE FUNDAMENTALS OF THE DASH DIET

The fundamentals of the DASH (Dietary Approaches to Stop Hypertension) diet are centered around specific principles and guidelines aimed at reducing blood pressure and promoting overall health. These fundamentals encompass various aspects of nutrition, lifestyle, and dietary patterns. Here are the key fundamentals of the DASH diet:

1. Emphasis on Nutrient-Dense Foods:

Fruits and Vegetables: Encourages the consumption of a variety of fruits and vegetables rich in vitamins, minerals, antioxidants, and fiber.

Whole Grains: Recommends whole grains over refined grains, providing more nutrients and fiber.

Lean Proteins: Advocates for lean sources of protein like poultry, fish, beans, nuts, and seeds, reducing saturated fat intake.

Low-Fat Dairy: Suggests low-fat or fat-free dairy products for essential nutrients with lower saturated fat content.

2. Sodium Reduction:

Limiting Sodium Intake: Emphasizes reducing sodium intake by choosing fresh foods over processed options, avoiding high-sodium condiments, and being mindful of added salt.

3. Balanced Macronutrients:

Portion Control: Promotes portion awareness without strict calorie counting, encouraging balanced meals.

Balanced Diet Composition: Focuses on a balance of carbohydrates, proteins, and healthy fats to support overall health and energy levels.

4. Moderation in Added Sugars and Sweets:

Reduced Sugary Foods: Advises moderation in consuming sweets, sugary beverages, and foods high in added sugars to control overall calorie intake.

5. Lifestyle Integration:

Physical Activity: Often integrated with recommendations for regular physical activity to complement dietary efforts.

Stress Management: Encourages stress reduction techniques as part of a holistic approach to health.

6. Personalization and Flexibility:

Adaptability: Can be tailored to individual dietary preferences, making it adaptable for various cultural and personal needs.

Long-Term Sustainability: Aims to be a sustainable, lifelong approach to eating rather than a short-term diet.

7. Evidence-Based Benefits:

Scientific Support: Backed by scientific research demonstrating its effectiveness in reducing blood pressure and improving overall health.

Versatility: Recognized not just for its blood pressure benefits but also for its potential in weight management and reducing the risk of chronic diseases.

The DASH diet's fundamentals revolve around a balanced intake of nutrient-dense foods, sodium reduction, portion control, moderation in added sugars, lifestyle integration, adaptability, and evidence-based benefits. By focusing on whole foods, healthy dietary patterns, and lifestyle modifications, the DASH diet aims to support heart health, manage blood pressure, and foster overall well-being, making it a versatile and sustainable dietary approach for improved health outcomes.

PORTION CONTROL AND RECOMMENDED SERVINGS

Portion control is a vital aspect of the DASH (Dietary Approaches to Stop Hypertension) diet, as it helps manage calorie intake and ensures a balanced consumption of various food groups. The diet provides recommended servings for different food groups, promoting portion awareness without strict calorie counting. Here's a breakdown of portion control and the recommended servings within the DASH diet:

Serving Sizes and Recommendations:

• Fruits:

Recommended Servings: Aim for 4-5 servings of fruits per day.

One Serving: Typically, one serving is equivalent to one medium-sized fruit (e.g., apple, orange), ½ cup of fresh, frozen, or canned fruits, or ¼ cup of dried fruits.

• Vegetables:

Recommended Servings: Aim for 4-5 servings of vegetables per day.

One Serving: One serving equals 1 cup of raw leafy vegetables, ½ cup of cooked vegetables, or ½ cup of vegetable juice.

• Grains (Whole Grains):

Recommended Servings: Aim for 6-8 servings of grains per day, with an emphasis on whole grains.

One Serving: One serving is equivalent to 1 slice of whole grain bread, ½ cup of cooked whole grain pasta, rice, or cereal, or 1 ounce of dry whole grains.

• Lean Proteins:

Recommended Servings: Aim for 2-3 servings of lean proteins per day.

One Serving: A serving typically equals 3 ounces of cooked lean meat, poultry, or fish, or ½ cup of cooked beans, lentils, or tofu.

• Low-Fat Dairy:

Recommended Servings: Aim for 2-3 servings of low-fat dairy products per day.

One Serving: One serving includes 1 cup of milk or yogurt, or 1.5 ounces of cheese (equivalent to 3-4 dice-sized cubes).

• Nuts, Seeds, and Legumes:

Recommended Servings: Incorporate nuts, seeds, or legumes a few times a week.

One Serving: A serving equals ⅓ cup of nuts, 2 tablespoons of seeds, or ½ cup of cooked beans or lentils.

• Fats and Oils:

Portion Control: While not strictly measured in servings, recommended intake involves moderation in using healthy fats and oils, such as using small amounts of olive oil or avocado.

Tips for Portion Control in the DASH Diet:

• Use Measuring Tools: Use measuring cups, spoons, or scales to accurately portion foods until you can estimate portions more easily.

• Visual Cues: Learn to estimate portion sizes using visual cues (e.g., a tennis ball for a medium fruit, a deck of cards for meat).

• Practice Balance: Strive for balanced meals by incorporating a variety of food groups in recommended servings.

• Mindful Eating: Pay attention to hunger cues and practice mindful eating to avoid overeating.

Portion control and adhering to the recommended servings of different food groups in the DASH diet are crucial for achieving a balanced and nutritious intake while managing calorie consumption. This approach ensures a varied diet rich in essential nutrients, supporting overall health and helping manage conditions like hypertension and weight.

THE FLEXIBILITY OF THE DIET AND HOW IT CAN BE ADAPTED FOR DIFFERENT PREFERENCES AND DIETARY NEEDS

The DASH (Dietary Approaches to Stop Hypertension) diet offers a considerable level of flexibility, making it adaptable to various preferences, dietary needs, cultural backgrounds, and individual health goals. This adaptability stems from the diet's focus on whole, nutrient-dense foods and its emphasis on balanced eating rather than strict rules or limitations. Here's how the DASH diet can be flexible and adapted for different preferences and dietary needs:

1. Food Substitutions:

Variety of Choices: The DASH diet provides multiple options within food groups, allowing individuals to choose foods they prefer while adhering to the diet's principles. For instance, different fruits, vegetables, grains, and proteins can be substituted based on personal taste.

2. Customizable Portions:

Portion Adaptation: While the diet recommends specific serving sizes, these can be adjusted based on individual calorie needs, activity levels, and health goals. For example, individuals requiring higher or lower calorie intake can adjust serving sizes accordingly.

3. Cultural Adaptation:

Incorporating Cultural Foods: The DASH diet allows for the inclusion of culturally specific foods within its framework. For instance, if certain traditional foods align with the DASH diet's principles, they can be incorporated into meals.

4. Allergy or Dietary Restrictions:

Substituting Allergens: Individuals with allergies or intolerances can make substitutions within food groups. For instance, dairy alternatives can replace milk products for those with lactose intolerance.

5. Vegetarian or Vegan Adaptation:

Plant-Based Emphasis: The DASH diet offers options for those following vegetarian or vegan diets by focusing on plant-based proteins like beans, lentils, nuts, and seeds.

6. Personalized Meal Planning:

Tailored Meal Plans: Individuals can create personalized meal plans based on their preferences and dietary needs while adhering to the DASH diet's fundamental principles.

Recipe Modification: Recipes can be modified to align with the DASH diet by making healthier ingredient choices and adjusting seasonings or cooking methods.

7. Long-Term Sustainability:

Lifestyle Integration: The flexibility of the DASH diet contributes to its long-term sustainability. It can be adopted as a lifestyle rather than a short-term diet, accommodating different preferences and evolving dietary needs over time.

The DASH diet's flexibility allows individuals to tailor their eating patterns while adhering to the fundamental principles of the diet. Its adaptability to diverse preferences and dietary needs makes it a versatile and sustainable approach to healthy eating. By providing a framework based on nutrient-dense foods, portion control, and balanced eating, the DASH diet can be customized to suit various cultural, lifestyle, and individual health requirements.

SCIENTIFIC EVIDENCE SUPPORTING THE EFFECTIVENESS OF THE DASH DIET FOR WEIGHT MANAGEMENT

The DASH (Dietary Approaches to Stop Hypertension) diet has been extensively studied for its impact on various health aspects, including weight management. Scientific evidence supports the effectiveness of the DASH diet in aiding weight loss and weight maintenance. Here's an overview of some key scientific studies supporting its efficacy:

1. Weight Loss Studies:

Comparison Studies: Research comparing the DASH diet to other dietary approaches, such as typical Western diets or higher-protein diets, has shown that the DASH diet can lead to significant weight loss.

Clinical Trials: Randomized controlled trials (RCTs) have demonstrated that individuals following the DASH diet experience weight loss over time compared to control groups.

2. Long-Term Weight Maintenance:

Sustainability: Studies have highlighted the long-term sustainability of the DASH diet for weight maintenance, suggesting that it's not only effective for initial weight loss but also for preventing weight regain.

Adherence and Lifestyle Changes: The DASH diet's emphasis on balanced nutrition and lifestyle changes contributes to its effectiveness in maintaining weight loss over an extended period.

3. Reduction in Body Mass Index (BMI) and Waist Circumference:

BMI Improvement: Several studies have indicated that adhering to the DASH diet results in reductions in body mass index (BMI), a measure of body fat, in both overweight and obese individuals.

Waist Circumference Reduction: The diet has been associated with decreases in waist circumference, a marker for abdominal obesity and related health risks.

4. Other Health Benefits Supporting Weight Management:

Blood Pressure Control: As the primary purpose of the DASH diet is to manage hypertension, studies have shown that its positive effects on blood pressure can indirectly contribute to weight management and cardiovascular health.

Improved Metabolic Markers: The diet's focus on nutrient-dense foods has been linked to improved metabolic markers, such as lower cholesterol levels and improved insulin sensitivity, which can aid weight loss and overall health.

Scientific evidence from various studies, including randomized controlled trials and comparative analyses, consistently demonstrates the efficacy of the DASH diet in promoting weight loss and supporting weight management. Its emphasis on whole, nutrient-dense foods, portion control, and a balanced approach to nutrition has been associated with favorable outcomes in reducing body weight, BMI, waist circumference, and improving overall metabolic health.

HOW TO SELECT DASH-FRIENDLY FOODS.

Selecting DASH-friendly foods involves choosing nutrient-rich options from various food groups while being mindful of sodium intake and portion sizes. Here's advice on selecting foods that align with the DASH (Dietary Approaches to Stop Hypertension) diet:

1. Fruits and Vegetables:

Variety: Choose a diverse range of colorful fruits and vegetables. Opt for fresh or frozen options without added sugars or sauces.

Fresh is Best: Prioritize fresh produce when possible, but frozen fruits and vegetables without added salt or sugar are also excellent choices.

2. Whole Grains:

Whole Grain Choices: Select whole grains like brown rice, quinoa, whole wheat bread, oats, barley, and whole grain pasta instead of refined grains.

Read Labels: Look for products labeled "100% whole grain" or "whole wheat" to ensure you're choosing truly whole grain options.

3. Lean Proteins:

Poultry and Fish: Opt for skinless poultry and fish like salmon, trout, and tuna. Grill, bake, or steam them instead of frying.

Plant-Based Proteins: Include beans, lentils, nuts, and seeds as sources of protein, which are low in saturated fat.

4. Low-Fat Dairy:

Low-Fat Choices: Choose low-fat or fat-free dairy products like milk, yogurt, and cheese to limit saturated fat intake.

Plain Options: Opt for plain varieties without added sugars or flavorings.

5. Nuts, Seeds, and Legumes:

Healthy Snacks: Incorporate unsalted nuts, seeds, or legumes as snacks or additions to salads and meals.

Portion Control: Be mindful of portion sizes as these foods are calorie-dense.

6. Healthy Fats and Oils:

Healthy Oil Choices: Use healthier oils like olive oil, canola oil, or avocado oil for cooking or as dressings.

Portion Moderation: Use oils in moderation due to their calorie density.

7. Sodium Awareness:

Fresh and Seasoned Foods: Choose fresh foods over processed items. When using canned foods, select low-sodium or no-salt-added options.

Herbs and Spices: Flavor meals with herbs, spices, lemon, or vinegar instead of salt to reduce sodium intake.

8. Limit Sweets and Added Sugars:

Moderation: Reduce intake of sweets, sugary beverages, and foods high in added sugars. Opt for healthier dessert choices or fresh fruits for sweetness.

9. Portion Control:

Mindful Eating: Pay attention to portion sizes, and use measuring tools if needed until you can estimate servings accurately.

Balanced Meals: Aim for balanced meals by including a variety of food groups in appropriate serving sizes.

Selecting DASH-friendly foods involves prioritizing whole, nutrient-dense options from all food groups, monitoring sodium intake, being mindful of portion sizes, and choosing healthier alternatives for added sugars and fats. Emphasize fresh produce, whole grains, lean proteins, and healthy fats while minimizing processed and high-sodium foods to align with the principles of the DASH diet.

HEALTHY COOKING METHODS TO RETAIN NUTRIENTS.

Healthy cooking methods can help retain nutrients in foods while minimizing the addition of unhealthy fats and excessive calories. Here are some cooking techniques that can help preserve nutrients:

1. Steaming:

Preserves Nutrients: Steaming is one of the best methods for retaining nutrients like vitamins and minerals, as it uses minimal water and doesn't expose the food to direct heat.

2. Boiling:

Nutrient Retention: Boiling in moderate amounts of water can help preserve nutrients, especially if you use the cooking liquid (e.g., for soups) where water-soluble vitamins may leach.

3. Grilling and Roasting:

Minimal Fat: Grilling and roasting with minimal added fats (like using a light coating of oil) can help retain nutrients while adding flavor through caramelization.

Use of Marinades: Preparing marinades with herbs, spices, and acidic components like vinegar or citrus can enhance flavors without compromising nutrients.

4. Stir-Frying and Sautéing:

Quick Cooking: Stir-frying and sautéing with small amounts of healthy oils (like olive oil or avocado oil) and high heat help retain nutrients due to the short cooking time.

Add Vegetables Later: Adding vegetables later in the cooking process can help retain their crunch and nutrients.

5. Microwave Cooking:

Short Cooking Time: Microwaving foods with minimal water and short cooking times can help retain nutrients, as it's a quick and efficient cooking method.

Cover Food: Covering food with a lid or microwave-safe wrap helps retain moisture and nutrients.

6. Minimal Processing:

Whole Food Preparation: Opt for minimal processing of foods to retain their natural nutrients. For instance, keeping vegetables and fruits whole or chopping them right before cooking.

7. Use of Cooking Liquids:

Retain Cooking Water: When possible, use cooking liquids (like broth or water) from boiled vegetables or grains in other recipes to retain water-soluble nutrients.

• Cutting Techniques: Cut vegetables in larger pieces to minimize surface area exposed to heat, preserving nutrients.

• Reduce Cooking Time: Aim to cook foods for the shortest time possible while still ensuring they are safe to eat.

• Avoid Overcooking: Overcooking can cause the loss of water-soluble vitamins like vitamin C and B-complex vitamins.

Utilizing cooking methods that involve minimal exposure to heat, minimal water usage, and shorter cooking times can help retain nutrients in foods. Combining these methods with the use of healthy fats, herbs, and spices enhances flavors while preserving the nutritional value of the ingredients.

THE IMPORTANCE OF PHYSICAL ACTIVITY ALONGSIDE DIET.

Physical activity plays a crucial role in overall health and well-being, complementing the benefits of a healthy diet. When combined with a nutritious diet, regular physical activity offers numerous advantages that contribute to a healthy lifestyle. Here's why physical activity is important alongside a balanced diet:

1. Weight Management:

Calorie Expenditure: Physical activity helps burn calories, supporting weight loss or weight maintenance when combined with a healthy diet.

Muscle Mass: Regular exercise helps preserve and build lean muscle mass, which can increase metabolism and aid in weight management.

2. Cardiovascular Health:

Heart Strength: Exercise strengthens the heart muscle, improves circulation, and lowers the risk of heart disease and stroke.

Blood Pressure: Regular physical activity can help manage blood pressure levels, complementing the effects of a heart-healthy diet like the DASH diet.

3. Improved Metabolism and Energy Levels:

Enhanced Metabolism: Exercise contributes to improved metabolism, helping the body process nutrients efficiently.

Increased Energy: Regular physical activity boosts energy levels, reducing fatigue and enhancing overall vitality.

4. Enhanced Mental Health:

Stress Reduction: Exercise triggers the release of endorphins, reducing stress, anxiety, and depression.

Improved Mood: Regular physical activity can positively impact mood and cognitive function, promoting overall mental well-being.

5. Bone Health and Strength:

Bone Density: Weight-bearing exercises help maintain bone density, reducing the risk of osteoporosis and fractures, especially in older adults.

Muscle Strength: Resistance training and weight-bearing exercises support muscle strength and flexibility.

6. Disease Prevention:

Reduced Risk of Chronic Diseases: Regular physical activity lowers the risk of various chronic conditions, including type 2 diabetes, certain cancers, and metabolic syndrome.

7. Better Sleep Quality:

Improved Sleep: Regular exercise promotes better sleep quality and duration, contributing to overall health and well-being.

8. Long-Term Health Benefits:

Lifestyle Habits: Physical activity is a key component of a healthy lifestyle, contributing to long-term health benefits when combined with a nutritious diet and other healthy habits.

Physical activity is an essential pillar of health that complements the benefits of a balanced diet. Incorporating regular exercise into daily routines not only aids in weight management but also enhances cardiovascular health, mental well-being, bone strength, disease prevention, and overall quality of life. When combined with a healthy diet like the DASH diet, regular physical activity forms a powerful foundation for optimal health and wellness throughout life.

EXERCISES AND ACTIVITIES THAT COMPLEMENT THE DIET PLAN

When complementing the DASH (Dietary Approaches to Stop Hypertension) diet with physical activity, it's essential to incorporate a variety of exercises that promote cardiovascular health, strength, flexibility, and overall well-being. Here are suitable exercises and activities that complement the DASH diet plan:

1. Aerobic/Cardiovascular Exercises:

• Brisk Walking: Walking is a simple yet effective aerobic exercise that can be done almost anywhere.

• Running or Jogging: Increases heart rate and offers cardiovascular benefits.

• Cycling: Riding a bike is a low-impact cardiovascular workout suitable for various fitness levels.

• Swimming: A full-body workout that is gentle on the joints, promoting cardiovascular health.

• Dancing: Engaging in dance routines or classes for a fun and effective cardiovascular workout.

• Aerobic Classes: Joining aerobic classes, Zumba, or step aerobics for variety and motivation.

2. Strength Training:

• Bodyweight Exercises: Incorporate exercises like squats, lunges, push-ups, and planks for muscle strength and endurance.

• Resistance Bands: Use resistance bands for strength training exercises targeting different muscle groups.

• Free Weights or Machines: Utilize free weights or gym machines for strength workouts.

3. Flexibility and Balance Exercises:

• Yoga: Practice yoga for improved flexibility, balance, and relaxation.

• Pilates: Focus on core strength, flexibility, and body awareness through Pilates exercises.

• Tai Chi: Engage in Tai Chi for balance, coordination, and relaxation.

4. High-Intensity Interval Training (HIIT):

• Short Bursts of Activity: Incorporate HIIT workouts involving short bursts of intense exercise followed by brief rest periods for cardiovascular benefits and calorie burning.

5. Outdoor Activities:

• Hiking: Enjoy hiking or trekking for a combination of cardiovascular exercise and nature appreciation.

• Gardening: Engage in gardening activities that involve physical movements, promoting flexibility and strength.

6. Mind-Body Exercises:

• Meditation: Incorporate mindfulness practices and meditation for stress reduction and mental well-being.

• Deep Breathing Exercises: Practice deep breathing techniques for relaxation and stress management.

Tips for Incorporating Exercise with the DASH Diet:

• Consistency: Aim for regular physical activity, striving for at least 150 minutes of moderate-intensity aerobic exercise or 75 minutes of vigorous-intensity exercise per week, as recommended by health guidelines.

• Variety: Incorporate a mix of aerobic, strength, flexibility, and balance exercises to ensure a well-rounded fitness routine.

• Gradual Progression: Start slowly and gradually increase the intensity and duration of workouts to prevent injury and maintain motivation.

Combining a range of cardiovascular exercises, strength training, flexibility workouts, and mind-body activities with the DASH diet supports overall health, enhances cardiovascular fitness, promotes strength and flexibility, reduces stress, and complements the dietary principles for optimal health and well-being.

COMMON CHALLENGES WHILE FOLLOWING THE DASH DIET AND HOW TO OVERCOME THEM.

While the DASH (Dietary Approaches to Stop Hypertension) diet offers numerous health benefits, individuals may face certain challenges when adopting this eating plan. Here are some common challenges and strategies to overcome them:

1. High Sodium Content in Processed Foods:

Challenge: Processed and packaged foods often contain high levels of sodium, which can be challenging to avoid.

Solution:

• Read Labels: Check food labels and choose low-sodium or no-salt-added options.

• Cook from Scratch: Prepare meals at home using fresh ingredients to control sodium content.

2. Adjusting to Different Eating Habits:

Challenge: Transitioning from previous eating habits to the DASH diet can be challenging.

Solution:

• Gradual Changes: Start by making small, gradual changes to your diet rather than attempting an abrupt overhaul.

• Experiment with Recipes: Explore new recipes that align with the DASH diet to keep meals interesting and flavorful.

3. Increased Grocery Expenses:

Challenge: Buying fresh produce and healthier food options might increase grocery expenses.

Solution:

• Budgeting and Planning: Plan meals in advance, create shopping lists, and look for seasonal produce or discounts to manage costs.

• Buy in Bulk: Consider buying non-perishable items or frozen fruits and vegetables in bulk to save money.

4. Time Constraints and Meal Preparation:

Challenge: Busy schedules can make it challenging to prepare meals following the DASH diet.

Solution:

• Meal Prep: Allocate time for meal prepping during weekends or free periods to have healthy meals ready for the week.

- Simple and Quick Recipes: Look for simple and quick-to-prepare recipes that align with the DASH diet.

5. Social Situations and Eating Out:

Challenge: Social gatherings or dining out may present challenges in sticking to the DASH diet.

Solution:

- Communication: Communicate your dietary preferences or restrictions to hosts or restaurant staff in advance.

- Smart Choices: Choose healthier options on the menu, such as grilled proteins, salads, or vegetable-based dishes.

6. Cravings for Unhealthy Foods:

Challenge: Cravings for high-fat or high-sugar foods may arise when transitioning to a healthier diet.

Solution:

- Substitute Healthier Options: Find healthier alternatives to satisfy cravings, such as fruit for sweets or nuts for snacks.

- Moderation: Allow occasional indulgences in moderation to prevent feelings of deprivation.

7. Staying Motivated:

Challenge: Staying motivated and consistent with the DASH diet can be difficult.

Solution:

• Set Realistic Goals: Set achievable goals and celebrate small successes along the way.

• Seek Support: Join online communities, find a diet buddy, or involve family members to support and motivate each other.

Overcoming challenges while following the DASH diet involves strategic planning, making gradual changes, seeking support, and being adaptable. By implementing these strategies, individuals can navigate common obstacles and successfully adopt and maintain a healthy eating pattern aligned with the principles of the DASH diet for better health outcomes.

TIPS FOR STAYING MOTIVATED AND ACCOUNTABLE.

Staying motivated and accountable while following a dietary plan like the DASH (Dietary Approaches to Stop Hypertension) diet is crucial for long-term success. Here are some effective tips to help maintain motivation and accountability:

1. Set Clear and Achievable Goals:

Specific Goals: Define clear, specific, and achievable goals related to your health, such as weight loss, improved blood pressure, or overall wellness.

Short-term and Long-term Goals: Break down larger goals into smaller, manageable milestones to track progress effectively.

2. Educate Yourself:

Understanding the Benefits: Learn about the benefits of the DASH diet for overall health and its impact on specific health goals like blood pressure management or weight loss.

Stay Informed: Continuously educate yourself about nutrition, healthy eating habits, and the importance of exercise in conjunction with the diet.

3. Keep a Food and Activity Journal:

Track Progress: Maintain a journal to log your daily food intake, physical activity, achievements, and challenges.

Accountability: Reviewing your journal helps stay accountable and provides insights into your habits and areas for improvement.

4. Find Support and Accountability Partners:

Join Support Groups: Engage with online communities, forums, or local support groups where you can share experiences, tips, and encouragement with others following the DASH diet.

Accountability Partners: Partner with a friend, family member, or a health coach to stay accountable and motivated together.

5. Reward Milestones and Celebrate Successes:

Incentivize Achievements: Set up rewards for reaching milestones or sticking to the diet consistently. Rewards can be non-food-related, such as treating yourself to a spa day or buying a new workout outfit.

Celebrate Successes: Celebrate your achievements, whether they're small or significant, to boost motivation and reinforce positive behavior.

6. Plan Ahead and Prepare:

Meal Planning: Plan your meals in advance, create grocery lists, and prepare healthy snacks to avoid impulsive, unhealthy choices.

Preparation is Key: Set aside time for meal prepping and organizing your kitchen to make following the DASH diet more convenient.

7. Stay Flexible and Learn from Setbacks:

Flexibility: Embrace flexibility and understand that occasional slip-ups are normal. Don't be too hard on yourself if you deviate from the plan occasionally.

Learn from Setbacks: Use setbacks as learning opportunities. Analyze what triggered the setback and devise strategies to overcome similar challenges in the future.

8. Visualize and Stay Positive:

Visualize Success: Picture the positive outcomes of achieving your health goals, and use visualization techniques to stay motivated.

Positive Self-talk: Practice positive self-talk and affirmations to maintain a constructive mindset.

Staying motivated and accountable while following the DASH diet requires commitment, planning, support, and a positive mindset. By setting realistic goals, tracking progress, seeking support, and maintaining a flexible approach, individuals can stay motivated and accountable on their journey toward better health and adherence to the DASH diet.

CHAPTER TWO

BREAKFAST RECIPES

Veggie Omelette with Whole Grain Toast

Ingredients:

• 2 eggs

• 1/4 cup diced bell peppers (any color)

• 1/4 cup diced onions

• 1/4 cup chopped spinach

• 1 tablespoon olive oil

• Salt and pepper to taste

• 2 slices of whole grain bread

Instructions:

1. In a bowl, beat the eggs and season with salt and pepper.

2. Heat olive oil in a non-stick skillet over medium heat. Add onions, bell peppers, and spinach. Sauté until vegetables are tender.

3. Pour beaten eggs over the sautéed vegetables in the skillet. Cook until the eggs are set, gently lifting the edges to let the uncooked eggs flow to the bottom.

4. Fold the omelette in half and slide it onto a plate. Toast the whole grain bread slices.

5. Serve the omelette with toasted whole grain bread on the side.

Greek Yogurt Parfait

Ingredients:

• 1 cup non-fat Greek yogurt

• 1/2 cup mixed fresh berries (strawberries, blueberries, raspberries)

• 2 tablespoons chopped nuts (almonds, walnuts)

• 1 tablespoon honey or maple syrup (optional)

Instructions:

1. In a glass or bowl, layer Greek yogurt, mixed berries, and chopped nuts.

2. Drizzle honey or maple syrup on top for added sweetness if desired.

Whole Grain Oatmeal with Fruit

Ingredients:

• 1/2 cup rolled oats

• 1 cup water or low-fat milk

• 1/2 teaspoon cinnamon

• 1/2 sliced banana

• Handful of berries (blueberries, raspberries)

• 1 tablespoon chopped nuts or seeds

Instructions:

1. In a saucepan, bring water or milk to a boil. Stir in the rolled oats and reduce heat to a simmer.

2. Cook for 5-7 minutes, stirring occasionally until oats are creamy and tender. Stir in cinnamon.

3. Transfer oatmeal to a bowl and top with sliced banana, berries, and chopped nuts or seeds.

Avocado Toast with Poached Egg

Ingredients:

• 1 slice of whole grain bread

• 1/2 ripe avocado, mashed

• 1 egg

• Salt and pepper to taste

• Optional toppings: chopped tomatoes, a sprinkle of feta cheese

Instructions:

1. Toast the whole grain bread until golden brown. Spread mashed avocado evenly on the toast.

2. Poach an egg in simmering water for about 3-4 minutes until the white is set but the yolk is still runny.

3. Carefully place the poached egg on top of the avocado toast.

4. Season with salt and pepper and add optional toppings if desired.

Ingredients:

• 1 cup spinach leaves

• 1/2 cup mixed berries (strawberries, blueberries, raspberries)

• 1/2 ripe banana

• 1/2 cup non-fat Greek yogurt

• 1/2 cup almond milk (unsweetened)

• 1 tablespoon chia seeds (optional)

Instructions:

1. Place spinach, mixed berries, banana, Greek yogurt, almond milk, and chia seeds in a blender.

2. Blend until smooth and creamy.

3. Pour into a glass and enjoy the nutritious smoothie.

Quinoa Breakfast Bowl

Ingredients:

• 1/2 cup cooked quinoa

- 1/4 cup sliced almonds

- 1/2 cup mixed berries (strawberries, blueberries)

- 1 tablespoon honey or maple syrup

- 1/4 teaspoon cinnamon

Instructions:

1. In a bowl, combine cooked quinoa, sliced almonds, mixed berries, honey or maple syrup, and cinnamon.

2. Stir well to mix all ingredients thoroughly.

3. Serve the quinoa mixture in a bowl and enjoy this hearty and protein-rich breakfast.

Veggie and Feta Egg Muffins

Ingredients:

- 4 eggs

- 1/4 cup diced bell peppers

- 1/4 cup chopped spinach

- 2 tablespoons crumbled feta cheese

- Salt and pepper to taste

Instructions:

1. Preheat the oven to 350°F (175°C) and grease a muffin tin.

2. In a bowl, whisk together eggs, diced bell peppers, chopped spinach, crumbled feta cheese, salt, and pepper.

3. Pour the egg mixture evenly into the muffin tin.

4. Bake for 15-18 minutes or until the egg muffins are set and slightly golden.

5. Remove from the oven, let them cool for a few minutes, and then remove the egg muffins from the tin. Serve warm.

Smoked Salmon and Avocado Toast

Ingredients:

- 1 slice of whole grain bread

- 2 ounces smoked salmon

- 1/4 ripe avocado, sliced

- 1 tablespoon low-fat cream cheese

- Fresh dill for garnish (optional)

Instructions:

1. Toast the whole grain bread until lightly crispy. Spread low-fat cream cheese on the toast.

2. Top with slices of smoked salmon and avocado. Garnish with fresh dill if desired and serve.

Banana-Berry Protein Pancakes

Ingredients:

• 1 ripe banana, mashed

• 2 eggs

• 1/4 teaspoon vanilla extract

• 1/4 cup mixed berries

• Cooking spray or oil for the pan

Instructions:

1. In a bowl, combine mashed banana, eggs, and vanilla extract. Mix until smooth.

2. Gently fold in the mixed berries into the batter.

3. Heat a non-stick skillet over medium heat and lightly coat it with cooking spray or oil.

4. Pour small portions of the batter onto the skillet to make pancakes. Cook until bubbles form on the surface, then flip and cook until golden brown on both sides.

5. Serve the pancakes warm with additional berries if desired.

Veggie Breakfast Burrito

Ingredients:

- 1 whole wheat tortilla

- 2 eggs, scrambled

- 1/4 cup black beans, drained and rinsed

- 1/4 cup diced tomatoes

- 2 tablespoons diced bell peppers

- 1 tablespoon chopped cilantro

- Salsa or hot sauce (optional)

Instructions:

1. Heat the whole wheat tortilla in a pan or microwave to soften it.

2. Fill the tortilla with scrambled eggs, black beans, diced tomatoes, diced bell peppers, and chopped cilantro.

3. Roll the tortilla tightly into a burrito.

4. Optionally, serve with salsa or hot sauce on the side for added flavor.

Spinach and Tomato Breakfast Frittata

Ingredients:

- 4 eggs

- 1 cup chopped spinach

- 1/2 cup diced tomatoes

- 1/4 cup diced onions

- 2 tablespoons grated Parmesan cheese

- 1 tablespoon olive oil

- Salt and pepper to taste

Instructions:

1. Preheat the oven to 350°F (175°C).

2. In a bowl, whisk eggs and season with salt and pepper.

3. Heat olive oil in an oven-safe skillet over medium heat. Sauté onions until translucent, then add spinach and tomatoes, cooking until spinach wilts.

4. Pour the whisked eggs evenly over the veggies in the skillet.

5. Sprinkle grated Parmesan cheese on top and cook on the stovetop for a few minutes until the edges start to set.

6. Transfer the skillet to the preheated oven and bake for about 10-12 minutes or until the frittata is set and golden. Slice and serve.

Chia Seed Pudding with Berries

Ingredients:

• 1/4 cup chia seeds

• 1 cup unsweetened almond milk

• 1 tablespoon honey or maple syrup (optional)

• 1/2 cup mixed berries (strawberries, blueberries, raspberries)

• Sliced almonds or shredded coconut for topping (optional)

Instructions:

1. In a bowl or jar, mix chia seeds, almond milk, and sweetener (if using). Stir well and refrigerate overnight or for at least 2-3 hours until it thickens.

2. Before serving, stir the chia seed mixture to ensure it's evenly thickened.

3. Top the chia seed pudding with mixed berries and optional sliced almonds or shredded coconut.

Mediterranean Breakfast Bowl

Ingredients:

• 1/2 cup cooked quinoa

• 2 tablespoons hummus

• 1/4 cup diced cucumbers

• 1/4 cup cherry tomatoes, halved

• 2 tablespoons chopped Kalamata olives

• 2 tablespoons crumbled feta cheese

• Fresh parsley for garnish (optional)

Instructions:

1. In a bowl, place cooked quinoa at the bottom.

2. Arrange hummus, diced cucumbers, cherry tomatoes, Kalamata olives, and crumbled feta cheese on top of the quinoa.

3. Garnish with fresh parsley if desired and serve.

Apple Cinnamon Overnight Oats

Ingredients:

- 1/2 cup rolled oats

- 1/2 cup unsweetened almond milk

- 1/2 medium apple, diced

- 1 tablespoon maple syrup or honey (optional)

- 1/4 teaspoon cinnamon

- Chopped nuts or raisins for topping (optional)

Instructions:

1. In a jar or bowl, combine rolled oats, almond milk, diced apple, sweetener (if using), and cinnamon. Mix well.

2. Cover and refrigerate overnight or for at least 4 hours.

3. Before serving, stir the overnight oats and top with chopped nuts or raisins if desired.

Ingredients:

- 1/2 cup firm tofu, crumbled

- 1/4 cup diced bell peppers

- 1/4 cup diced onions

- 1/2 cup chopped spinach

- 1 teaspoon olive oil

- 1/4 teaspoon turmeric (for color)

- Salt and pepper to taste

Instructions:

1. Heat olive oil in a skillet over medium heat. Sauté onions and bell peppers until soft.

2. Add crumbled tofu, turmeric, chopped spinach, salt, and pepper. Cook for a few minutes until heated through and spinach wilts.

3. Serve the tofu and veggie scramble warm.

Whole Grain Breakfast Burrito

Ingredients:

- 1 whole grain tortilla

- 2 eggs, scrambled

- 1/4 cup black beans, drained and rinsed

- 2 tablespoons diced bell peppers

- 2 tablespoons diced tomatoes

- 1 tablespoon chopped cilantro

- 2 tablespoons shredded low-fat cheese

- Salsa or hot sauce (optional)

Instructions:

1. Heat the whole grain tortilla in a pan or microwave to warm it up.

2. Fill the tortilla with scrambled eggs, black beans, bell peppers, tomatoes, cilantro, and shredded cheese.

3. Roll the tortilla into a burrito shape.

4. Optionally, serve with salsa or hot sauce on the side.

Banana Peanut Butter Smoothie Bowl

Ingredients:

• 1 ripe banana

• 2 tablespoons natural peanut butter

• 1/2 cup non-fat Greek yogurt

• 1/4 cup unsweetened almond milk

• 1 tablespoon chia seeds (optional)

• Toppings: Sliced banana, granola, chopped nuts

Instructions:

1. In a blender, combine ripe banana, peanut butter, Greek yogurt, almond milk, and chia seeds (if using). Blend until smooth.

2. Pour the smoothie into a bowl.

3. Top with sliced banana, granola, and chopped nuts for added texture and flavor.

Ingredients:

- 1 small sweet potato, diced

- 1/2 cup diced bell peppers

- 1/4 cup diced onions

- 1 cup chopped spinach

- 2 eggs

- 1 tablespoon olive oil

- Salt, pepper, and paprika to taste

Instructions:

1. Heat olive oil in a skillet over medium heat. Add diced sweet potatoes and cook until they start to soften.

2. Add diced bell peppers and onions to the skillet. Cook until vegetables are tender.

3. Stir in chopped spinach and season with salt, pepper, and paprika.

4. Create two wells in the hash mixture and crack an egg into each well.

5. Cover the skillet and cook until the eggs are cooked to your desired consistency. Serve the veggie breakfast hash warm.

Berry Almond Chia Pudding

Ingredients:

- 2 tablespoons chia seeds

- 1/2 cup unsweetened almond milk

- 1/2 cup mixed berries (strawberries, blueberries)

- 1 tablespoon sliced almonds

- 1 tablespoon honey or maple syrup (optional)

Instructions:

1. In a bowl or jar, mix chia seeds and almond milk. Stir well and refrigerate for at least 2 hours or overnight until it thickens.

2. Before serving, layer the chia pudding with mixed berries and sliced almonds.

3. Drizzle honey or maple syrup on top if desired.

Ingredients:

• 4 eggs

• 1/4 cup chopped spinach

• 1/4 cup diced tomatoes

• 2 tablespoons chopped black olives

• 2 tablespoons crumbled feta cheese

• Salt and pepper to taste

Instructions:

1. Preheat the oven to 350°F (175°C) and grease a muffin tin.

2. In a bowl, whisk eggs and season with salt and pepper.

3. Divide chopped spinach, diced tomatoes, black olives, and crumbled feta cheese among the muffin tin cups.

4. Pour the whisked eggs evenly over the vegetable mixture in the muffin tin cups.

5. Bake for about 15-18 minutes or until the egg muffin cups are set and slightly golden.

6. Allow them to cool for a few minutes before removing them from the tin. Serve warm.

Ingredients:

- 1/2 cup cooked quinoa

- 1/2 cup unsweetened almond milk

- 1/4 teaspoon cinnamon

- 1/4 teaspoon vanilla extract

- 1 tablespoon chopped nuts (walnuts, almonds)

- 1 tablespoon dried fruits (raisins, cranberries)

- Optional sweetener: honey or maple syrup

Instructions:

1. In a saucepan, combine cooked quinoa, almond milk, cinnamon, and vanilla extract. Heat over medium-low heat, stirring occasionally.

2. Once heated through and thickened to desired consistency, remove from heat.

3. Stir in chopped nuts, dried fruits, and sweetener if desired.

4. Serve the quinoa porridge warm.

Ingredients:

• 4 eggs

• 1/4 cup chopped bell peppers

• 1/4 cup chopped spinach

• 2 tablespoons crumbled goat cheese

• 1 tablespoon chopped fresh herbs (parsley, basil)

• Salt and pepper to taste

Instructions:

1. Preheat the oven to 350°F (175°C) and grease a muffin tin.

2. In a bowl, whisk eggs and season with salt and pepper.

3. Divide chopped bell peppers, spinach, crumbled goat cheese, and fresh herbs among the muffin tin cups.

4. Pour the whisked eggs evenly over the vegetable mixture in the muffin tin cups.

5. Bake for about 15-18 minutes or until the frittata cups are set and slightly golden.

6. Allow them to cool for a few minutes before removing them from the tin. Serve warm or at room temperature.

Open-Faced Smoked Salmon Sandwich

Ingredients:

• 1 slice of whole grain bread

• 2 ounces smoked salmon

• 2 tablespoons low-fat cream cheese

• 2 slices of cucumber

• Fresh dill for garnish

• Lemon wedges for serving (optional)

Instructions:

1. Toast the whole grain bread until lightly crispy. Spread low-fat cream cheese on the toast.

2. Layer slices of smoked salmon and cucumber on top. Garnish with fresh dill.

3. Serve with lemon wedges for squeezing over the salmon if desired.

Berry and Greek Yogurt Parfait

Ingredients:

- 1/2 cup non-fat Greek yogurt

- 1/4 cup mixed berries (strawberries, blueberries)

- 2 tablespoons granola

- 1 tablespoon honey or maple syrup (optional)

Instructions:

1. In a glass or bowl, layer Greek yogurt, mixed berries, and granola.

2. Drizzle honey or maple syrup on top for added sweetness if desired.

Spinach and Mushroom Breakfast Wrap

Ingredients:

• 1 whole grain tortilla

• 2 eggs, scrambled

• 1/4 cup chopped spinach

• 1/4 cup sliced mushrooms

• 1 tablespoon shredded low-fat cheese

• Salt and pepper to taste

Instructions:

1. Heat the whole grain tortilla in a pan or microwave to warm it up.

2. Fill the tortilla with scrambled eggs, chopped spinach, sliced mushrooms, and shredded cheese. Roll the tortilla into a wrap.

3. Optionally, heat it in a pan for a few minutes to slightly crisp up the tortilla.

4. Serve the breakfast wrap warm.

Grilled Lemon Herb Chicken with Quinoa Salad

Ingredients:

Grilled Lemon Herb Chicken:

- 2 boneless, skinless chicken breasts

- 2 tablespoons olive oil

- 2 cloves garlic, minced

- 1 tablespoon fresh lemon juice

- 1 teaspoon dried thyme

- Salt and pepper to taste

Quinoa Salad:

- 1 cup cooked quinoa

- 1/2 cup cherry tomatoes, halved

- 1/4 cup chopped cucumber

- 2 tablespoons chopped fresh parsley

- 2 tablespoons chopped red onion

- 2 tablespoons feta cheese (optional)

• 2 tablespoons lemon vinaigrette (olive oil, lemon juice, Dijon mustard)

Instructions:

1. In a bowl, mix olive oil, minced garlic, lemon juice, dried thyme, salt, and pepper. Marinate chicken breasts in the mixture for at least 30 minutes.

2. Preheat grill or grill pan over medium-high heat. Grill chicken breasts for 6-8 minutes per side until cooked through.

3. For the quinoa salad, combine cooked quinoa, cherry tomatoes, cucumber, parsley, red onion, feta cheese, and lemon vinaigrette. Toss gently to combine.

4. Serve the grilled lemon herb chicken alongside the quinoa salad.

Mediterranean Chickpea Salad

Ingredients:

• 1 can (15 oz) chickpeas, drained and rinsed

• 1/2 cup diced cucumber

• 1/2 cup cherry tomatoes, halved

- 1/4 cup chopped red onion

- 1/4 cup chopped fresh parsley

- 2 tablespoons chopped Kalamata olives

- 2 tablespoons crumbled feta cheese (optional)

- Lemon juice, olive oil, salt, and pepper for dressing

Instructions:

1. In a bowl, combine chickpeas, diced cucumber, cherry tomatoes, red onion, parsley, Kalamata olives, and feta cheese.

2. Drizzle with lemon juice and olive oil. Season with salt and pepper. Toss gently to coat.

3. Serve the Mediterranean chickpea salad as a refreshing and protein-rich lunch option.

Turkey and Avocado Wrap

Ingredients:

- 1 whole grain wrap or tortilla

- 3 ounces sliced turkey breast

- 1/4 avocado, sliced

- 1/4 cup shredded lettuce

- 1/4 cup sliced bell peppers

- 1 tablespoon hummus or low-fat cream cheese

Instructions:

1. Lay the whole grain wrap or tortilla on a flat surface.

2. Spread hummus or low-fat cream cheese evenly on the wrap.

3. Layer sliced turkey breast, avocado slices, shredded lettuce, and sliced bell peppers.

4. Roll the wrap tightly and slice it in half diagonally for serving.

Veggie and Tuna Salad Bowl

Ingredients:

- 1 can (5 oz) tuna in water, drained

- 1 cup mixed greens (spinach, lettuce)

- 1/2 cup chopped cucumber

- 1/2 cup diced tomatoes

- 1/4 cup sliced red onion

- 1/4 cup shredded carrots

- 2 tablespoons balsamic vinaigrette

Instructions:

1. In a bowl, combine mixed greens, chopped cucumber, diced tomatoes, red onion, and shredded carrots. Top with flaked tuna.

2. Drizzle with balsamic vinaigrette dressing.

3. Toss gently to combine all ingredients and enjoy the veggie and tuna salad bowl.

Vegetable Stir-Fry with Brown Rice

Ingredients:

- 1 cup mixed vegetables (broccoli, bell peppers, snap peas)

- 1/2 cup sliced mushrooms

- 1/4 cup diced tofu or cooked chicken breast (optional)

- 1 tablespoon low-sodium soy sauce

- 1 tablespoon olive oil

- 1/2 teaspoon minced garlic

- Cooked brown rice

Instructions:

1. Heat olive oil in a skillet or wok over medium-high heat. Add minced garlic and sauté for a minute.

2. Add mixed vegetables, sliced mushrooms, and tofu or chicken if using. Stir-fry for 5-6 minutes until vegetables are tender-crisp.

3. Add low-sodium soy sauce and toss the vegetables to coat evenly.

4. Serve the vegetable stir-fry over cooked brown rice.

Baked Salmon with Quinoa and Steamed Vegetables

Ingredients:

Baked Salmon:

- 2 salmon fillets

- 1 tablespoon olive oil

- 1 teaspoon lemon zest

- 1 teaspoon dried dill

• Salt and pepper to taste

Quinoa and Steamed Vegetables:

• 1 cup cooked quinoa

• 1 cup mixed steamed vegetables (broccoli, carrots, bell peppers)

• 1 tablespoon chopped fresh parsley

• Lemon wedges for serving (optional)

Instructions:

1. Preheat the oven to 375°F (190°C).

2. Place the salmon fillets on a baking sheet lined with parchment paper.

3. Drizzle olive oil over the salmon and sprinkle with lemon zest, dried dill, salt, and pepper.

4. Bake for 12-15 minutes or until the salmon is cooked through.

5. In a bowl, combine cooked quinoa, mixed steamed vegetables, and chopped parsley.

6. Serve the baked salmon alongside the quinoa and steamed vegetables. Garnish with lemon wedges if desired.

Greek Chicken Salad

Ingredients:

- 2 cups chopped cooked chicken breast

- 1 cup chopped cucumbers

- 1 cup cherry tomatoes, halved

- 1/4 cup sliced red onion

- 1/4 cup sliced Kalamata olives

- 2 tablespoons crumbled feta cheese

- 2 tablespoons chopped fresh parsley

- Lemon vinaigrette (olive oil, lemon juice, oregano)

Instructions:

1. In a large bowl, combine chopped chicken breast, cucumbers, cherry tomatoes, red onion, Kalamata olives, feta cheese, and chopped parsley.

2. Drizzle with lemon vinaigrette dressing and toss gently to coat.

3. Serve the Greek chicken salad chilled.

Ingredients:

- 1 cup dried green lentils

- 4 cups low-sodium vegetable or chicken broth

- 1 cup diced carrots

- 1 cup diced celery

- 1 cup diced onions

- 2 cloves garlic, minced

- 1 teaspoon dried thyme

- Salt and pepper to taste

- Chopped fresh parsley for garnish

Instructions:

1. Rinse lentils under cold water and drain.

2. In a large pot, combine lentils, broth, carrots, celery, onions, garlic, dried thyme, salt, and pepper.

3. Bring to a boil, then reduce heat to low and simmer for 25-30 minutes or until lentils and vegetables are tender.

4. Adjust seasoning if needed and garnish with chopped fresh parsley before serving.

Whole Grain Pasta Primavera

Ingredients:

• 2 cups whole grain pasta (penne or spaghetti)

• 1 cup mixed vegetables (broccoli, bell peppers, zucchini)

• 2 cloves garlic, minced

• 2 tablespoons olive oil

• 1/4 cup grated Parmesan cheese

• 1 tablespoon chopped fresh basil

• Salt and pepper to taste

Instructions:

1. Cook whole grain pasta according to package instructions. Drain and set aside.

2. In a pan, heat olive oil over medium heat. Add minced garlic and sauté for a minute.

3. Add mixed vegetables and cook until tender-crisp. Toss cooked pasta with the vegetable mixture.

4. Sprinkle grated Parmesan cheese and chopped basil over the pasta. Season with salt and pepper, toss gently, and serve.

Black Bean and Quinoa Stuffed Bell Peppers

Ingredients:

• 4 bell peppers, halved and seeds removed

• 1 cup cooked quinoa

• 1 can (15 oz) black beans, drained and rinsed

• 1 cup diced tomatoes

• 1/2 cup corn kernels

• 1/4 cup chopped cilantro

• 1 teaspoon ground cumin

• 1/2 teaspoon chili powder

• Salt and pepper to taste

• Shredded low-fat cheese for topping (optional)

Instructions:

1. Preheat the oven to 375°F (190°C).

2. In a bowl, mix cooked quinoa, black beans, diced tomatoes, corn kernels, chopped cilantro, ground cumin, chili powder, salt, and pepper.

3. Spoon the quinoa and black bean mixture into each bell pepper half.

4. Place stuffed bell peppers in a baking dish. Cover with foil and bake for 25-30 minutes.

5. Optionally, top with shredded low-fat cheese in the last 5 minutes of baking.

6. Serve the black bean and quinoa stuffed bell peppers hot.

Quinoa Salad with Chickpeas and Veggies

Ingredients:

• 1 cup cooked quinoa

• 1 can (15 oz) chickpeas, drained and rinsed

• 1 cup diced cucumbers

• 1 cup cherry tomatoes, halved

- 1/4 cup diced red onions

- 1/4 cup chopped fresh parsley

- 2 tablespoons olive oil

- 2 tablespoons lemon juice

- Salt and pepper to taste

Instructions:

1. In a large bowl, combine cooked quinoa, chickpeas, diced cucumbers, cherry tomatoes, red onions, and chopped parsley.

2. In a small bowl, whisk together olive oil, lemon juice, salt, and pepper.

3. Drizzle the dressing over the salad and toss gently to combine.

4. Serve the quinoa salad chilled or at room temperature.

Turkey and Veggie Lettuce Wraps

Ingredients:

- 8 large lettuce leaves (such as iceberg or butter lettuce)

- 1/2 pound cooked turkey breast, sliced

- 1/2 cup shredded carrots

- 1/2 cup sliced bell peppers

- 1/4 cup thinly sliced cucumbers

- 1/4 cup hummus or low-fat Greek yogurt

- Fresh herbs for garnish (optional)

Instructions:

1. Lay out the lettuce leaves on a clean surface. Spread hummus or Greek yogurt onto each lettuce leaf.

2. Divide the sliced turkey, shredded carrots, bell peppers, and cucumbers among the lettuce leaves. Garnish with fresh herbs if desired.

3. Roll the lettuce leaves to form wraps and secure them with toothpicks if needed.

Veggie and Tofu Stir-Fry

Ingredients:

- 1 block (14 oz) extra-firm tofu, pressed and cubed

- 2 cups mixed vegetables (broccoli, bell peppers, snap peas)

- 2 cloves garlic, minced

- 2 tablespoons low-sodium soy sauce

- 1 tablespoon sesame oil

- 1 tablespoon rice vinegar

- Cooked brown rice or quinoa for serving

Instructions:

1. Heat sesame oil in a skillet or wok over medium-high heat.

2. Add minced garlic and cubed tofu. Sauté until tofu is golden brown. Add mixed vegetables to the skillet and stir-fry until tender-crisp.

3. In a small bowl, mix low-sodium soy sauce and rice vinegar. Pour the mixture over the tofu and vegetables.

4. Stir well to combine and cook for an additional minute.

5. Serve the vegetable and tofu stir-fry over cooked brown rice or quinoa.

Mediterranean Chickpea Wraps

Ingredients:

- 4 whole grain wraps or tortillas

- 1 can (15 oz) chickpeas, drained and rinsed

- 1 cup chopped cucumbers

- 1 cup diced tomatoes

- 1/4 cup sliced red onions

- 2 tablespoons chopped fresh parsley

- 2 tablespoons hummus

- Lemon wedges for serving (optional)

Instructions:

1. Lay out the whole grain wraps or tortillas on a flat surface.

2. Spread hummus evenly on each wrap.

3. Divide chickpeas, chopped cucumbers, diced tomatoes, red onions, and chopped parsley among the wraps.

4. Squeeze fresh lemon juice over the fillings if desired. Roll the wraps tightly, cut in half, and serve.

Tuna and Avocado Lettuce Wraps

Ingredients:

• 1 can (5 oz) tuna in water, drained

• 1 ripe avocado, mashed

• 1/4 cup diced red onions

• 2 tablespoons chopped celery

• 1 tablespoon lemon juice

• 8 large lettuce leaves (such as Boston or Bibb lettuce)

Instructions:

1. In a bowl, mix drained tuna, mashed avocado, diced red onions, chopped celery, and lemon juice.

2. Lay out the lettuce leaves on a clean surface.

3. Spoon the tuna and avocado mixture onto each lettuce leaf.

4. Roll the lettuce leaves to form wraps and serve.

Veggie and Hummus Wrap

Ingredients:

- 4 whole grain wraps or tortillas

- 1/2 cup hummus

- 1 cup mixed greens

- 1/2 cup sliced bell peppers

- 1/2 cup shredded carrots

- 1/4 cup sliced cucumbers

- Fresh herbs for garnish (optional)

Instructions:

1. Lay out the whole grain wraps or tortillas on a flat surface. Spread hummus evenly on each wrap.

2. Divide mixed greens, sliced bell peppers, shredded carrots, and sliced cucumbers among the wraps. Garnish with fresh herbs if desired.

3. Roll the wraps tightly, cut in half, and serve.

Eggplant and Zucchini Ratatouille

Ingredients:

- 1 large eggplant, diced

- 2 zucchinis, diced

- 1 onion, chopped

- 2 cloves garlic, minced

- 2 cups diced tomatoes (canned or fresh)

- 1 tablespoon olive oil

- 1 teaspoon dried thyme

- Salt and pepper to taste

- Chopped fresh basil for garnish

Instructions:

1. Heat olive oil in a large skillet or pot over medium heat.

2. Add chopped onions and minced garlic. Sauté until onions are translucent.

3. Add diced eggplant and zucchinis. Cook for 5-7 minutes until slightly softened. Stir in diced tomatoes, dried thyme, salt, and pepper.

4. Cover and simmer for 20-25 minutes until vegetables are tender.

5. Garnish with chopped fresh basil before serving.

Lemon Herb Grilled Salmon Salad

Ingredients:

• 2 salmon fillets

• 4 cups mixed greens

• 1/2 cup cherry tomatoes, halved

• 1/4 cup sliced cucumber

• 1/4 cup sliced red onions

• 2 tablespoons chopped fresh dill

• 2 tablespoons olive oil

• 1 tablespoon lemon juice

• Salt and pepper to taste

Instructions:

1. Preheat the grill to medium-high heat. Season the salmon fillets with salt, pepper, and a drizzle of olive oil.

2. Grill the salmon for about 4-5 minutes per side or until cooked through.

3. In a large bowl, toss mixed greens, cherry tomatoes, sliced cucumber, red onions, and chopped fresh dill.

4. In a separate small bowl, whisk together olive oil, lemon juice, salt, and pepper for the dressing.

5. Place grilled salmon on top of the salad and drizzle with the lemon herb dressing.

Turkey and Quinoa Stuffed Bell Peppers

Ingredients:

• 4 bell peppers, halved and seeds removed

• 1 cup cooked quinoa

• 1/2 pound ground turkey

• 1 cup diced tomatoes

• 1/4 cup chopped onions

• 1/4 cup shredded low-fat cheese

• 1 teaspoon Italian seasoning

• Salt and pepper to taste

Instructions:

1. Preheat the oven to 375°F (190°C).

2. In a skillet over medium heat, cook ground turkey until browned. Add diced tomatoes, chopped onions, Italian seasoning, salt, and pepper. Cook for 5 minutes.

3. Stir in cooked quinoa and shredded low-fat cheese into the turkey mixture. Spoon the mixture into each bell pepper half.

4. Place stuffed bell peppers in a baking dish. Cover with foil and bake for 25-30 minutes.

5. Serve the turkey and quinoa stuffed bell peppers hot.

Veggie and Brown Rice Stir-Fry

Ingredients:

• 2 cups cooked brown rice

• 2 cups mixed vegetables (broccoli, bell peppers, carrots)

• 1 cup tofu or chicken, diced (optional)

• 2 tablespoons low-sodium soy sauce

• 1 tablespoon sesame oil

• 1 tablespoon rice vinegar

• 1 teaspoon minced garlic

• 1 teaspoon grated ginger

• Chopped green onions for garnish

Instructions:

1. Heat sesame oil in a large skillet or wok over medium-high heat.

2. Add minced garlic and grated ginger. Sauté for a minute.

3. Add mixed vegetables and tofu or chicken (if using) to the skillet. Stir-fry until vegetables are tender-crisp.

4. In a small bowl, mix low-sodium soy sauce and rice vinegar. Pour the mixture over the stir-fry and toss to coat.

5. Add cooked brown rice to the skillet and stir-fry for an additional 2-3 minutes.

6. Garnish with chopped green onions before serving.

Lentil and Vegetable Wrap

Ingredients:

• 4 whole grain wraps or tortillas

- 1 cup cooked lentils

- 1 cup mixed vegetables (bell peppers, spinach, carrots)

- 1/4 cup diced red onions

- 2 tablespoons hummus or Greek yogurt

- Fresh cilantro or parsley for garnish

Instructions:

1. Lay out the whole grain wraps or tortillas on a flat surface.

2. Spread hummus or Greek yogurt evenly on each wrap.

3. Divide cooked lentils, mixed vegetables, and diced red onions among the wraps. Garnish with fresh cilantro or parsley.

4. Roll the wraps tightly, cut in half, and serve.

Shrimp and Vegetable Stir-Fry

Ingredients:

- 1 pound shrimp, peeled and deveined

- 2 cups mixed vegetables (broccoli, bell peppers, snow peas)

- 2 cloves garlic, minced

- 1 tablespoon low-sodium soy sauce

- 1 tablespoon hoisin sauce

- 1 teaspoon sesame oil

- 1 tablespoon olive oil

- Cooked brown rice for serving

Instructions:

1. Heat olive oil in a large skillet or wok over medium-high heat.

2. Add minced garlic and stir-fry for 30 seconds. Add shrimp to the skillet and cook until pink and opaque.

3. Add mixed vegetables and continue stir-frying until tender-crisp.

4. In a small bowl, mix low-sodium soy sauce, hoisin sauce, and sesame oil. Pour the sauce over the shrimp and vegetables.

5. Stir well to combine and cook for an additional minute.

6. Serve the shrimp and vegetable stir-fry over cooked brown rice.

Greek Quinoa Salad with Chicken

Ingredients:

• 2 grilled chicken breasts, sliced

• 2 cups cooked quinoa

• 1 cup diced cucumbers

• 1 cup cherry tomatoes, halved

• 1/4 cup diced red onions

• 1/4 cup chopped Kalamata olives

• 2 tablespoons chopped fresh parsley

• 2 tablespoons olive oil

• 2 tablespoons red wine vinegar

• Salt and pepper to taste

• Crumbled feta cheese for topping (optional)

Instructions:

1. In a large bowl, combine cooked quinoa, diced cucumbers, cherry tomatoes, red onions, Kalamata olives, and chopped parsley.

2. Add grilled chicken slices to the salad.

3. In a small bowl, whisk together olive oil, red wine vinegar, salt, and pepper for the dressing.

4. Drizzle the dressing over the salad and toss gently. Top with crumbled feta cheese before serving.

Veggie and Hummus Plate

Ingredients:

• 1 cup assorted raw vegetables (carrots, cucumbers, bell peppers)

• 1/4 cup hummus

• 1/4 cup whole grain pita wedges

• 2 tablespoons mixed nuts (almonds, walnuts)

Instructions:

1. Arrange assorted raw vegetables on a plate. Serve with hummus for dipping.

2. Place whole grain pita wedges and mixed nuts on the plate as sides.

3. Enjoy as a light and nutritious lunch option.

Turkey Medallions with Tomato Salad

Ingredients:

- 2 tablespoons olive oil

- 1 tablespoon red wine vinegar

- 1/2 teaspoon sugar

- 1/4 teaspoon dried oregano

- 1/4 teaspoon salt

- 1 medium green pepper, coarsely chopped

- 1 celery rib, coarsely chopped

- 1/4 cup chopped red onion

- 1 tablespoon thinly sliced fresh basil

- 3 medium tomatoes

Turkey:

- 1 large egg

- 2 tablespoons lemon juice

- 1 cup panko bread crumbs

- 1/2 cup grated Parmesan cheese

- 1/2 cup finely chopped walnuts

- 1 teaspoon lemon-pepper seasoning

- 1 package (20 ounces) turkey breast tenderloins

- 1/4 teaspoon salt

- 1/4 teaspoon pepper

- 3 tablespoons olive oil

- Additional fresh basil

Instructions:

1. Whisk together first 5 ingredients. Stir in green pepper, celery, onion and basil. Cut tomatoes into wedges; cut wedges in half. Stir into pepper mixture.

2. In a shallow bowl, whisk together egg and lemon juice. In another shallow bowl, toss bread crumbs with cheese, walnuts and lemon pepper.

3. Cut tenderloins crosswise into 1-in. slices; flatten slices with a meat mallet to 1/2-in. thickness. Sprinkle with salt and pepper. Dip in egg mixture, then in crumb mixture, patting to adhere.

4. In a large skillet, heat 1 tablespoon oil over medium-high heat. Add a third of the turkey; cook until golden brown, 2-3 minutes per side. Repeat twice with remaining oil and turkey. Serve with tomato mixture; sprinkle with basil.

Strawberry-Blue Cheese Steak Salad

Ingredients:

- 1 beef top sirloin steak (3/4 inch thick and 1 pound)

- 1/2 teaspoon salt

- 1/4 teaspoon pepper

- 2 teaspoons olive oil

- 2 tablespoons lime juice

Salad:

- 1 bunch romaine, torn (about 10 cups)

- 2 cups fresh strawberries, halved

- 1/4 cup thinly sliced red onion

- 1/4 cup crumbled blue cheese

- 1/4 cup chopped walnuts, toasted

• Reduced-fat balsamic vinaigrette

Instructions:

1. Season steak with salt and pepper. In a large skillet, heat oil over medium heat. Add steak; cook 5-7 minutes on each side until meat reaches desired doneness (for medium-rare, a thermometer should read 135°; medium, 140°; medium-well, 145°). Remove from pan; let stand 5 minutes. Cut steak into bite-sized strips; toss with lime juice.

2. On a platter, combine romaine, strawberries and onion; top with steak. Sprinkle with cheese and walnuts. Serve with vinaigrette.

Black Bean & Sweet Potato Rice Bowls

Ingredients:

• 3/4 cup uncooked long grain rice

• 1/4 teaspoon garlic salt

• 1-1/2 cups water

• 3 tablespoons olive oil, divided

• 1 large sweet potato, peeled and diced

- 1 medium red onion, finely chopped

- 4 cups chopped fresh kale (tough stems removed)

- 1 can (15 ounces) black beans, rinsed and drained

- 2 tablespoons sweet chili sauce

- Optional: Lime wedges and additional sweet chili sauce

Instructions:

1. Place rice, garlic salt and water in a large saucepan; bring to a boil. Reduce heat; simmer, covered, until water is absorbed and rice is tender, 15-20 minutes. Remove from heat; let stand 5 minutes.

2. Meanwhile, in a large skillet, heat 2 tablespoons oil over medium-high heat; saute sweet potato 8 minutes. Add onion; cook and stir until potato is tender, 4-6 minutes. Add kale; cook and stir until tender, 3-5 minutes. Stir in beans; heat through.

3. Gently stir 2 tablespoons chili sauce and remaining oil into rice; add to potato mixture. If desired, serve with lime wedges and additional chili sauce.

Ingredients:

- 1/3 cup orange juice

- 3 tablespoons cider vinegar

- 1-1/2 teaspoons Dijon mustard

- 1-1/2 teaspoons honey

- 1 tablespoon minced fresh tarragon

Salad:

- 4 teaspoons canola oil, divided

- 1 cup fresh or frozen corn

- 1 pound uncooked shrimp (26-30 per pound), peeled and deveined

- 1/2 teaspoon lemon-pepper seasoning

- 1/4 teaspoon salt

- 8 cups torn mixed salad greens

- 2 medium nectarines, cut into 1-inch pieces

- 1 cup grape tomatoes, halved

• 1/2 cup finely chopped red onion

Instructions:

1. In a small bowl, whisk orange juice, vinegar, mustard and honey until blended. Stir in tarragon.

2. In a large skillet, heat 1 teaspoon oil over medium-high heat. Add corn; cook and stir 1-2 minutes or until crisp-tender. Remove from pan.

3. Sprinkle shrimp with lemon pepper and salt. In the same skillet, heat remaining oil over medium-high heat. Add shrimp; cook and stir 3-4 minutes or until shrimp turn pink. Stir in corn.

4. In a large bowl, combine remaining ingredients. Drizzle with 1/3 cup dressing and toss to coat. Divide mixture among four plates. Top with shrimp mixture; drizzle with remaining dressing. Serve immediately.

Pork Chops with Tomato Curry

Ingredients:

• 4 teaspoons butter, divided

• 6 boneless pork loin chops (6 ounces each)

• 1 small onion, finely chopped

- 3 medium apples, thinly sliced (about 5 cups)

- 1 can (28 ounces) whole tomatoes, undrained

- 4 teaspoons sugar

- 2 teaspoons curry powder

- 1/2 teaspoon salt

- 1/2 teaspoon chili powder

- 4 cups hot cooked brown rice

- 2 tablespoons toasted slivered almonds, optional

Instructions:

1. In a 6-qt. stockpot, heat 2 teaspoons butter over medium-high heat. Brown pork chops in batches. Remove from pan.

2. In same pan, heat remaining butter over medium heat. Add onion; cook and stir 2-3 minutes or until tender. Stir in apples, tomatoes, sugar, curry powder, salt and chili powder. Bring to a boil, stirring to break up tomatoes.

3. Return chops to pan. Reduce heat; simmer, uncovered, 5 minutes. Turn chops; cook 3-5 minutes longer or until a thermometer inserted in pork reads 145°. Let stand 5 minutes before serving. Serve with rice and, if desired, sprinkle with almonds.

Thai Chicken Pasta Skillet

Ingredients:

• 6 ounces uncooked whole wheat spaghetti

• 2 teaspoons canola oil

• 1 package (10 ounces) fresh sugar snap peas, trimmed and cut diagonally into thin strips

• 2 cups julienned carrots (about 8 ounces)

• 2 cups shredded cooked chicken

• 1 cup Thai peanut sauce

• 1 medium cucumber, halved lengthwise, seeded and sliced diagonally

• Chopped fresh cilantro, optional

Instructions:

1. Cook spaghetti according to package directions; drain.

2. Meanwhile, in a large skillet, heat oil over medium-high heat. Add snap peas and carrots; stir-fry 6-8 minutes or until crisp-tender. Add chicken, peanut sauce and spaghetti; heat through, tossing to combine.

3. Transfer to a serving plate. Top with cucumber and, if desired, cilantro.

Ingredients

• 6 medium zucchini (about 8 ounces each)

• 1 pound Italian turkey sausage links, casings removed

• 2 medium tomatoes, seeded and chopped

• 1 cup panko bread crumbs

• 1/3 cup grated Parmesan cheese

• 1/3 cup minced fresh parsley

• 2 tablespoons minced fresh oregano or 2 teaspoons dried oregano

• 2 tablespoons minced fresh basil or 2 teaspoons dried basil

• 1/4 teaspoon pepper

• 3/4 cup shredded part-skim mozzarella cheese

• Additional minced fresh parsley, optional

Instructions:

1. Preheat oven to 350°. Cut each zucchini lengthwise in half. Scoop out flesh, leaving a 1/4-in. shell; chop flesh.

2. Place zucchini shells in a large microwave-safe dish. In batches, microwave, covered, on high 2-3 minutes or until crisp-tender.

3. In a large skillet, cook sausage and zucchini flesh over medium heat 6-8 minutes or until sausage is no longer pink, breaking sausage into crumbles; drain. Stir in tomatoes, bread crumbs, Parmesan cheese, herbs and pepper. Spoon into zucchini shells.

4. Place in 2 ungreased 13x9-in. baking dishes. Bake, covered, 15-20 minutes or until zucchini is tender. Sprinkle with mozzarella cheese.

5. Bake, uncovered, 5-8 minutes longer or until cheese is melted. If desired, sprinkle with additional minced parsley.

Spiced Salmon

Ingredients:

- 2 tablespoons brown sugar

- 1 tablespoon soy sauce

- 1 tablespoon butter, melted

- 1 tablespoon olive oil

- 1/2 teaspoon garlic powder

- 1/2 teaspoon ground mustard

- 1/2 teaspoon paprika

- 1/2 teaspoon pepper

- 1/4 teaspoon dill weed

- Dash salt

- Dash dried tarragon

- Dash cayenne pepper

- 1 salmon fillet (2 pounds)

Instructions:

1. Mix all ingredients except salmon; brush over salmon.

2. Place salmon, skin side down, on an oiled grill rack or on a lightly oiled baking sheet. Grill, covered, over medium heat or broil 4 in. from heat until fish just begins to flake easily with a fork, 10-15 minutes.

Tomato Green Bean Soup

Ingredients:

- 1 cup chopped onion

- 1 cup chopped carrots

- 2 teaspoons butter

- 6 cups reduced-sodium chicken or vegetable broth

- 1 pound fresh green beans, cut into 1-inch pieces

- 1 garlic clove, minced

- 3 cups diced fresh tomatoes

- 1/4 cup minced fresh basil or 1 tablespoon dried basil

- 1/2 teaspoon salt

- 1/4 teaspoon pepper

Instructions:

1. In a large saucepan, saute onion and carrots in butter for 5 minutes. Stir in the broth, beans and garlic; bring to a boil. Reduce heat; cover and simmer for 20 minutes or until vegetables are tender.

2. Stir in the tomatoes, basil, salt and pepper. Cover and simmer 5 minutes longer.

Peppered Sole

Ingredients:

• 2 tablespoons butter

• 2 cups sliced fresh mushrooms

• 2 garlic cloves, minced

• 4 sole fillets (4 ounces each)

• 1/4 teaspoon paprika

• 1/4 teaspoon lemon-pepper seasoning

• 1/8 teaspoon cayenne pepper

• 1 medium tomato, chopped

• 2 green onions, thinly sliced

Instructions:

1. In a large skillet, heat butter over medium-high heat. Add mushrooms; cook and stir until tender. Add garlic; cook 1 minute longer. Place fillets over mushrooms. Sprinkle with paprika, lemon pepper and cayenne.

2. Cook, covered, over medium heat 5-10 minutes or until fish just begins to flake easily with a fork. Sprinkle with tomato and green onions.

Shrimp Orzo with Feta

Ingredients:

• 1-1/4 cups uncooked whole wheat orzo pasta

• 2 tablespoons olive oil

• 2 garlic cloves, minced

• 2 medium tomatoes, chopped

• 2 tablespoons lemon juice

• 1-1/4 pounds uncooked shrimp (26-30 per pound), peeled and deveined

• 2 tablespoons minced fresh cilantro

• 1/4 teaspoon pepper

- 1/2 cup crumbled feta cheese

Instructions:

1. Cook orzo according to package directions. Meanwhile, in a large skillet, heat oil over medium heat. Add garlic; cook and stir 1 minute. Add tomatoes and lemon juice. Bring to a boil. Stir in shrimp. Reduce heat; simmer, uncovered, until shrimp turn pink, 4-5 minutes.

2. Drain orzo. Add orzo, cilantro and pepper to shrimp mixture; heat through. Sprinkle with feta cheese.

Citrus-Herb Pork Roast

Ingredients:

- 1 boneless pork sirloin roast (3 to 4 pounds)

- 1 teaspoon dried oregano

- 1/2 teaspoon ground ginger

- 1/2 teaspoon pepper

- 2 medium onions, cut into thin wedges

- 1 cup plus 3 tablespoons orange juice, divided

- 1 tablespoon sugar

* 1 tablespoon white grapefruit juice

* 1 tablespoon steak sauce

* 1 tablespoon reduced-sodium soy sauce

* 1 teaspoon grated orange zest

* 1/2 teaspoon salt

* 3 tablespoons cornstarch

* Hot cooked egg noodles

* Minced fresh oregano, optional

Instructions:

1. Cut roast in half. In a small bowl, combine the oregano, ginger and pepper; rub over pork. In a large skillet coated with cooking spray, brown roast on all sides. Transfer to a 4-qt. slow cooker; add onions.

2. In a small bowl, combine 1 cup orange juice, sugar, grapefruit juice, steak sauce and soy sauce; pour over top.

3. Cover and cook on low for 4-5 hours or until meat is tender. Remove meat and onions to a serving platter; keep warm.

4. Skim fat from cooking juices; transfer to a small saucepan. Add orange zest and salt. Bring to a boil. Combine cornstarch and the remaining orange juice until smooth. Gradually stir into the pan.

5. Bring to a boil; cook and stir for 2 minutes or until thickened. Serve with pork and noodles; if desired, sprinkle with fresh oregano.

Grilled Tilapia with Pineapple Salsa

Ingredients:

- 2 cups cubed fresh pineapple

- 2 green onions, chopped

- 1/4 cup finely chopped green pepper

- 1/4 cup minced fresh cilantro

- 4 teaspoons plus 2 tablespoons lime juice, divided

- 1/8 teaspoon plus 1/4 teaspoon salt, divided

- Dash cayenne pepper

- 1 tablespoon canola oil

- 8 tilapia fillets (4 ounces each)

- 1/8 teaspoon pepper

Instructions:

1. For salsa, in a small bowl, combine pineapple, green onions, green pepper, cilantro, 4 teaspoons lime juice, 1/8 teaspoon salt and cayenne. Refrigerate until serving.

2. Mix oil and remaining lime juice; drizzle over fillets. Sprinkle with pepper and remaining salt.

3. Grill fish, covered, on an oiled rack over medium heat or broil 4 in. from heat until fish just begins to flake easily with a fork, 2-3 minutes on each side. Serve with salsa.

Peppered Tuna Kabobs

Ingredients:

- 1/2 cup frozen corn, thawed

- 4 green onions, chopped

- 1 jalapeno pepper, seeded and chopped

- 2 tablespoons coarsely chopped fresh parsley

- 2 tablespoons lime juice

- 1 pound tuna steaks, cut into 1-inch cubes

- 1 teaspoon coarsely ground pepper

- 2 large sweet red peppers, cut into 2x1-inch pieces

- 1 medium mango, peeled and cut into 1-inch cubes

Instructions:

1. For salsa, in a small bowl, combine the first five ingredients; set aside.

2. Rub tuna with pepper. On four metal or soaked wooden skewers, alternately thread red peppers, tuna and mango.

3. Place skewers on greased grill rack. Cook, covered, over medium heat, turning occasionally, until tuna is slightly pink in center (medium-rare) and peppers are tender, 10-12 minutes. Serve with salsa.

Cherry-Chicken Lettuce Wraps

Ingredients:

- 3/4 pound boneless skinless chicken breasts, cut into 3/4-inch cubes

- 1 teaspoon ground ginger

- 1/4 teaspoon salt

* 1/4 teaspoon pepper

* 2 teaspoons olive oil

* 1-1/2 cups shredded carrots

* 1-1/4 cups coarsely chopped pitted fresh sweet cherries

* 4 green onions, chopped

* 1/3 cup coarsely chopped almonds

* 2 tablespoons rice vinegar

* 2 tablespoons reduced-sodium teriyaki sauce

* 1 tablespoon honey

* 8 Bibb or Boston lettuce leaves

Instructions:

1. Sprinkle chicken with ginger, salt and pepper. In a large nonstick skillet, heat oil over medium-high heat. Add chicken; cook and stir 3-5 minutes or until no longer pink.

2. Remove from heat. Stir in carrots, cherries, green onions and almonds. In a small bowl, mix vinegar, teriyaki sauce and honey; stir into chicken mixture. Divide among lettuce leaves; fold lettuce over filling.

Ingredients:

- 6 large eggs

- 3 large egg whites

- 1/4 cup salsa

- 1 tablespoon minced fresh parsley

- 1/4 teaspoon salt

- 1/4 teaspoon pepper

- 1 tablespoon olive oil

- 1/3 cup finely chopped green pepper

- 1/3 cup finely chopped sweet red pepper

- 3 green onions, finely chopped

- 2 garlic cloves, minced

- 1 cup canned black beans, rinsed and drained

- 1/2 cup shredded white cheddar cheese

- Optional toppings: Minced fresh cilantro, sliced ripe olives and additional salsa

Instructions:

1. Preheat broiler. In a large bowl, whisk the first 6 ingredients until blended.

2. In a 10-in. ovenproof skillet, heat oil over medium-high heat. Add peppers and green onions; cook and stir 3-4 minutes or until peppers are tender.

3. Add garlic; cook 1 minute longer. Stir in beans. Reduce heat to medium; stir in egg mixture. Cook, uncovered, 4-6 minutes or until nearly set. Sprinkle with cheese.

4. Broil 3-4 in. from heat 3-4 minutes or until light golden brown and eggs are completely set. Let stand 5 minutes. Cut into wedges. Serve with toppings as desired.

Thai-Style Cobb Salad

Ingredients:

- 1 bunch romaine, torn

- 2 cups shredded rotisserie chicken

- 3 hard-boiled large eggs, coarsely chopped

- 1 medium ripe avocado, peeled and thinly sliced

- 1 medium carrot, shredded

- 1 medium sweet red pepper, julienned

- 1 cup fresh snow peas, halved

- 1/2 cup unsalted peanuts

- 1/4 cup fresh cilantro leaves

- 3/4 cup Asian toasted sesame salad dressing

- 2 tablespoons creamy peanut butter

Instructions:

1. Place romaine on a large serving platter. Arrange chicken, eggs, avocado, vegetables and peanuts over romaine; sprinkle with cilantro.

2. In a small bowl, whisk salad dressing and peanut butter until smooth. Serve with salad.

Turkey and Vegetable Barley Soup

Ingredients:

- 1 tablespoon canola oil

- 5 medium carrots, chopped

- 1 medium onion, chopped

- 2/3 cup quick-cooking barley

- 6 cups reduced-sodium chicken broth

- 2 cups cubed cooked turkey breast

- 2 cups fresh baby spinach

- 1/2 teaspoon pepper

Instructions:

1. In a large saucepan, heat oil over medium-high heat. Add carrots and onion; cook and stir until carrots are crisp-tender, 4-5 minutes.

2. Stir in barley and broth; bring to a boil. Reduce heat; simmer, covered, until carrots and barley are tender, 10-15 minutes. Stir in turkey, spinach and pepper; heat through.

Grilled Southwestern Steak Salad

Ingredients:

- 1 beef top sirloin steak (1 inch thick and 3/4 pound)

- 1/4 teaspoon salt

- 1/4 teaspoon ground cumin

- 1/4 teaspoon pepper

- 3 poblano peppers, halved and seeded

- 2 large ears sweet corn, husks removed

- 1 large sweet onion, cut into 1/2-inch rings

- 1 tablespoon olive oil

- 2 cups uncooked multigrain bow tie pasta

- 2 large tomatoes

Dressing:

- 1/4 cup lime juice

- 1 tablespoon olive oil

- 1/4 teaspoon salt

- 1/4 teaspoon ground cumin

- 1/4 teaspoon pepper

- 1/3 cup chopped fresh cilantro

Instructions:

1. Rub steak with salt, cumin and pepper. Brush poblano peppers, corn and onion with oil. Grill steak, covered, over medium heat or broil 4 in. from heat 6-8 minutes on each side or until meat reaches desired doneness (for medium-rare, a thermometer should read 135°; medium, 140°; medium-well, 145°). Grill vegetables, covered, 8-10 minutes or until crisp-tender, turning occasionally.

2. Cook pasta according to package directions. Meanwhile, cut corn from cob; coarsely chop peppers, onion and tomatoes. Transfer vegetables to a large bowl. In a small bowl, whisk lime juice, oil, salt, cumin and pepper until blended; stir in cilantro.

3. Drain pasta; add to vegetable mixture. Drizzle with dressing; toss to coat. Cut steak into thin slices; add to salad.

Cabbage Roll Skillet

Ingredients:

• 1 can (28 ounces) whole plum tomatoes, undrained

• 1 pound extra-lean ground beef (95% lean)

• 1 large onion, chopped

• 1 can (8 ounces) tomato sauce

- 2 tablespoons cider vinegar

- 1 tablespoon brown sugar

- 1 teaspoon dried oregano

- 1 teaspoon dried thyme

- 1/2 teaspoon pepper

- 1 small head cabbage, thinly sliced (about 6 cups)

- 1 medium green pepper, cut into thin strips

- 4 cups hot cooked brown rice

Instructions:

1. Drain tomatoes, reserving liquid; coarsely chop tomatoes. In a large nonstick skillet, cook beef and onion over medium-high heat 6-8 minutes or until beef is no longer pink, breaking up beef into crumbles. Stir in tomato sauce, vinegar, brown sugar, seasonings, chopped tomatoes and reserved liquid.

2. Add cabbage and pepper; cook, covered, 6 minutes, stirring occasionally. Cook, uncovered, 6-8 minutes or until cabbage is tender. Serve with rice.

Warm Rice & Pintos Salad

Ingredients:

• 1 tablespoon olive oil

• 1 cup frozen corn

• 1 small onion, chopped

• 2 garlic cloves, minced

• 1-1/2 teaspoons chili powder

• 1-1/2 teaspoons ground cumin

• 1 can (15 ounces) pinto beans, rinsed and drained

• 1 package (8.8 ounces) ready-to-serve brown rice

• 1 can (4 ounces) chopped green chiles

• 1/2 cup salsa

• 1/4 cup chopped fresh cilantro

• 1 bunch romaine, quartered lengthwise through the core

• 1/4 cup finely shredded cheddar cheese

Instructions:

1. In a large skillet, heat oil over medium-high heat. Add corn and onion; cook and stir 4-5 minutes or until onion is tender. Stir in garlic, chili powder and cumin; cook and stir 1 minute longer.

2. Add beans, rice, green chiles, salsa and cilantro; heat through, stirring occasionally.

3. Serve over romaine wedges. Sprinkle with cheese.

Roasted Sweet Potato & Chickpea Pitas

Ingredients:

• 2 medium sweet potatoes (about 1-1/4 pounds), peeled and cubed

• 2 cans (15 ounces each) chickpeas or garbanzo beans, rinsed and drained

• 1 medium red onion, chopped

• 3 tablespoons canola oil, divided

• 2 teaspoons garam masala

• 1/2 teaspoon salt, divided

• 2 garlic cloves, minced

• 1 cup plain Greek yogurt

- 1 tablespoon lemon juice

- 1 teaspoon ground cumin

- 2 cups arugula or baby spinach

- 12 whole wheat pita pocket halves, warmed

- 1/4 cup minced fresh cilantro

Instructions:

1. Preheat oven to 400°. Place potatoes in a large microwave-safe bowl; microwave, covered, on high 5 minutes. Stir in chickpeas and onion; toss with 2 tablespoons oil, garam masala and 1/4 teaspoon salt.

2. Spread into a 15x10x1-in. pan. Roast until potatoes are tender, about 15 minutes. Cool slightly.

3. Place garlic and remaining 1 Tbsp. oil in a small microwave-safe bowl; microwave on high until garlic is lightly browned, 1 to 1-1/2 minutes. Stir in yogurt, lemon juice, cumin and remaining 1/4 tsp. salt.

4. Toss potato mixture with arugula. Spoon into pitas; top with sauce and cilantro.

Ingredients:

• 3 cups uncooked whole wheat elbow macaroni (about 12 ounces)

• 1 can (15 ounces) cannellini beans, rinsed and drained

• 2 cups cherry tomatoes, halved

• 1 cup fresh or frozen corn, thawed

• 1/2 cup finely chopped red onion

• 1/2 cup part-skim ricotta cheese

• 1/4 cup grated Parmesan cheese

• 2 tablespoons minced fresh basil or 2 teaspoons dried basil

• 1 tablespoon olive oil

• 3 garlic cloves, minced

• 1 teaspoon salt

• 1 teaspoon minced fresh rosemary or 1/2 teaspoon dried rosemary, crushed

• 1/2 teaspoon pepper

• 3 cups arugula or baby spinach

• Chopped fresh parsley, optional

Instructions:

1. Cook pasta according to package directions. Drain and rinse with cold water; drain well.

2. In a large bowl, combine beans, tomatoes, corn, onion, ricotta and Parmesan cheeses, basil, oil, garlic, salt, rosemary and pepper. Stir in pasta.

3. Add arugula; toss gently to combine. If desired, sprinkle with parsley. Serve immediately.

Pesto Corn Salad with Shrimp

Ingredients:

• 4 medium ears sweet corn, husked

• 1/2 cup packed fresh basil leaves

• 1/4 cup olive oil

• 1/2 teaspoon salt, divided

• 1-1/2 cups cherry tomatoes, halved

• 1/8 teaspoon pepper

- 1 medium ripe avocado, peeled and chopped

- 1 pound uncooked shrimp (31-40 per pound), peeled and deveined

Instructions:

1. In a pot of boiling water, cook corn until tender, about 5 minutes. Drain; cool slightly. Meanwhile, in a food processor, pulse basil, oil and 1/4 teaspoon salt until blended.

2. Cut corn from cob and place in a bowl. Stir in tomatoes, pepper and remaining 1/4 teaspoon salt. Add avocado and 2 tablespoons basil mixture; toss gently to combine.

3. Thread shrimp onto metal or soaked wooden skewers; brush with remaining basil mixture. Grill, covered, over medium heat until shrimp turn pink, 2-4 minutes per side. Remove shrimp from skewers; serve with corn mixture.

Salmon with Horseradish Pistachio Crust

Ingredients:

- 6 salmon fillets (4 ounces each)

- 1/3 cup sour cream

- 2/3 cup dry bread crumbs

- 2/3 cup chopped pistachios

- 1/2 cup minced shallots

- 2 tablespoons olive oil

- 1 to 2 tablespoons prepared horseradish

- 1 tablespoon snipped fresh dill or 1 teaspoon dill weed

- 1/2 teaspoon grated lemon or orange zest

- 1/4 teaspoon crushed red pepper flakes

- 1 garlic clove, minced

Instructions:

1. Preheat oven to 350°. Place salmon, skin side down, in an ungreased 15x10x1-in. baking pan. Spread sour cream over each fillet. Combine remaining ingredients.

2. Pat crumb-nut mixture onto tops of salmon fillets, pressing to help coating adhere. Bake until fish just begins to flake easily with a fork, 12-15 minutes.

Southwest Shredded Pork Salad

Ingredients:

- 1 boneless pork loin roast (3 to 4 pounds)

- 1-1/2 cups apple cider or juice

- 1 can (4 ounces) chopped green chiles, drained

- 3 garlic cloves, minced

- 1-1/2 teaspoons salt

- 1-1/2 teaspoons hot pepper sauce

- 1 teaspoon chili powder

- 1 teaspoon pepper

- 1/2 teaspoon ground cumin

- 1/2 teaspoon dried oregano

- 12 cups torn mixed salad greens

- 1 can (15 ounces) black beans, rinsed and drained

- 2 medium tomatoes, chopped

- 1 small red onion, chopped

- 1 cup fresh or frozen corn

- 1 cup crumbled Cotija or shredded part-skim mozzarella cheese

• Salad dressing of your choice

Instructions:

1. Place pork in a 5- or 6-qt. slow cooker. In a small bowl, mix cider, green chiles, garlic, salt, pepper sauce, chili powder, pepper, cumin and oregano; pour over pork. Cook, covered, on low 6-8 hours or until meat is tender.

2. Remove roast from slow cooker; discard cooking juices. Shred pork with 2 forks. Arrange salad greens on a large serving platter. Top with pork, black beans, tomatoes, onion, corn and cheese. Serve with salad dressing.

White Wine Garlic Chicken

Ingredients:

• 4 boneless skinless chicken breast halves (6 ounces each)

• 1/2 teaspoon salt

• 1/4 teaspoon pepper

• 1 tablespoon olive oil

• 2 cups sliced baby portobello mushrooms (about 6 ounces)

- 1 medium onion, chopped

- 2 garlic cloves, minced

- 1/2 cup dry white wine or reduced-sodium chicken broth

Instructions:

1. Pound chicken breasts with a meat mallet to 1/2-in. thickness; sprinkle with salt and pepper. In a large skillet, heat oil over medium heat; cook chicken until no longer pink, 5-6 minutes per side. Remove from pan; keep warm.

2. Add mushrooms and onion to pan; cook and stir over medium-high heat until tender and lightly browned, 2-3 minutes. Add garlic; cook and stir 30 seconds.

3. Add wine; bring to a boil, stirring to loosen browned bits from pan. Cook until liquid is slightly reduced, 1-2 minutes; serve over chicken.

Maple-Roasted Chicken Thighs with Sweet Potato Wedges and Brussels Sprouts

Ingredients:

- 2 tablespoons pure maple syrup

- 4 teaspoons olive oil

- 1 tablespoon snipped fresh thyme

- ½ teaspoon salt

- ½ teaspoon black pepper

- 1 pound sweet potatoes, peeled and cut into 1-inch wedges

- 1 pound Brussels sprouts, trimmed and halved

- Nonstick cooking spray

- 4 bone-in chicken thighs, skinned

- 3 tablespoons snipped dried cranberries

- 3 tablespoons chopped pecans, toasted

Instructions:

1. Preheat oven to 425 degrees F. In a small bowl combine maple syrup, 1 tsp. of the oil, the thyme, 1/4 tsp. of the salt, and 1/4 tsp. of the pepper.

2. In a large bowl combine sweet potatoes and Brussels sprouts. Drizzle with the remaining 1 tbsp. oil and sprinkle with the remaining 1/4 tsp. salt and 1/4 tsp. pepper; toss to coat.

3. Line a 15x10-inch baking pan with foil. Heat the prepared pan in oven 5 minutes. Remove pan from oven and coat with cooking spray. Arrange chicken, meaty sides down, in center of pan. Arrange vegetables around chicken. Roast 15 minutes.

4. Turn chicken and vegetables; brush with maple syrup mixture. Roast 15 minutes more or until chicken is done (at least 175 degrees F) and potatoes are tender. Serve topped with pecans and cranberries.

Spicy Shrimp, Vegetable & Couscous Bowls

Ingredients:

- 1 ½ cups whole-wheat pearl couscous

- 1 small red bell pepper, chopped

- ½ cup snow peas, trimmed and sliced

- 3 tablespoons sliced fresh basil, divided

- 3 tablespoons sliced fresh mint, divided

- 1 cup chopped fresh cilantro

- 2 tablespoons lime juice

- 1 tablespoon rice vinegar

• 1 tablespoon water

• 1 ½ teaspoons sambal oelek

• 1 ½ teaspoons grated fresh ginger

• 1 large clove garlic, crushed and peeled

• ½ teaspoon ground pepper, divided

• ⅛ teaspoon salt

• 5 tablespoons grapeseed oil, divided

• 1 pound large raw shrimp (16-20 count), peeled and deveined

Directions

1. Cook couscous according to package directions. Drain, rinse and place in a large bowl. Add bell pepper, snow peas and 2 tablespoons each basil and mint.

2. Meanwhile, combine cilantro, lime juice, vinegar, water, sambal oelek, ginger, garlic, 1/4 teaspoon pepper and salt in a blender. Blend until smooth. With the motor running, slowly drizzle in 4 tablespoons oil. Set aside 2 tablespoons of the dressing. Toss the remaining dressing with the couscous and vegetables to coat.

3. Heat the remaining 1 tablespoon oil in a large skillet over high heat. Pat shrimp dry and sprinkle with the

remaining 1/4 teaspoon pepper. Add to the pan and cook, flipping once, until just cooked through, about 2 minutes per side. Serve the shrimp and couscous mixture with the reserved 2 tablespoons dressing and the remaining 1 tablespoon each basil and mint.

Sheet-Pan Harissa Chicken and Vegetables

Ingredients:

- 4 cups white or purple cauliflower florets

- 4 cups sliced red, orange and/or yellow bell peppers

- 3 tablespoons extra-virgin olive oil, divided

- ¼ teaspoon kosher salt, plus 1/2 teaspoon, divided

- 2 teaspoons harissa paste, plus 1/2 teaspoon, divided

- 1 teaspoon brown sugar

- 1 clove garlic, minced

- 2 8-ounce boneless, skinless chicken breasts

- ½ cup whole-milk plain Greek yogurt

- 1 teaspoon lemon zest

- 2 tablespoons lemon juice

- 1 teaspoon minced fresh mint

- 1 teaspoon minced fresh parsley

- ⅛ teaspoon ground pepper

Instructions:

1. Preheat oven to 400 degrees F. Toss cauliflower and peppers with 2 tablespoons oil and 1/4 teaspoon salt in a large bowl. Spread in a single layer on a large rimmed baking sheet; roast for 15 minutes.

2. Meanwhile, combine 2 teaspoons harissa paste, brown sugar, garlic and the remaining 1 tablespoon oil and 1/2 teaspoon salt in a small bowl. Rub chicken all over with the harissa mixture. Stir the vegetables, then add the chicken to the pan. Roast until a thermometer inserted into the thickest part of the chicken registers 165 degrees F, about 20 minutes.

3. Combine yogurt, the remaining 1/2 teaspoon harissa paste, lemon zest and juice, mint, parsley and pepper in a small bowl. Drizzle the sauce over the chicken and vegetables or serve on the side for dipping.

Walnut-Rosemary Crusted Salmon

Ingredients:

- 2 teaspoons Dijon mustard

- 1 clove garlic, minced

- ¼ teaspoon lemon zest

- 1 teaspoon lemon juice

- 1 teaspoon chopped fresh rosemary

- ½ teaspoon honey

- ½ teaspoon kosher salt

- ¼ teaspoon crushed red pepper

- 3 tablespoons panko breadcrumbs

- 3 tablespoons finely chopped walnuts

- 1 teaspoon extra-virgin olive oil

- 1 (1 pound) skinless salmon fillet, fresh or frozen

- Olive oil cooking spray

- Chopped fresh parsley and lemon wedges for garnish

Instructions:

1. Preheat oven to 425 degrees F. Line a large rimmed baking sheet with parchment paper.

2. Combine mustard, garlic, lemon zest, lemon juice, rosemary, honey, salt and crushed red pepper in a small bowl. Combine panko, walnuts and oil in another small bowl.

3. Place salmon on the prepared baking sheet. Spread the mustard mixture over the fish and sprinkle with the panko mixture, pressing to adhere. Lightly coat with cooking spray.

4. Bake until the fish flakes easily with a fork, about 8 to 12 minutes, depending on thickness.

5. Sprinkle with parsley and serve with lemon wedges, if desired.

One-Pot Garlicky Shrimp and Spinach

Ingredients

- 3 tablespoons extra-virgin olive oil, divided

- 6 medium cloves garlic, sliced, divided

- 1 pound spinach

- ¼ teaspoon salt plus 1/8 teaspoon, divided

- 1 tablespoon lemon juice

- 1 pound shrimp (21-30 count), peeled and deveined

- ¼ teaspoon crushed red pepper

- 1 tablespoon finely chopped fresh parsley

- 1 ½ teaspoons lemon zest

Instructions:

1. Heat 1 tablespoon oil in a large pot over medium heat. Add half the garlic and cook until beginning to brown, 1 to 2 minutes. Add spinach and 1/4 teaspoon salt and toss to coat.

2. Cook, stirring once or twice, until mostly wilted, 3 to 5 minutes. Remove from heat and stir in lemon juice. Transfer to a bowl and keep warm.

3. Increase heat to medium-high and add the remaining 2 tablespoons oil to the pot. Add the remaining garlic and cook until beginning to brown, 1 to 2 minutes.

4. Add shrimp, crushed red pepper and the remaining 1/8 teaspoon salt; cook, stirring, until the shrimp are just cooked through, 3 to 5 minutes more. Serve the shrimp over the spinach, sprinkled with lemon zest and parsley.

Roasted Salmon with Smoky Chickpeas and Greens

Ingredients:

• 2 tablespoons extra-virgin olive oil, divided

• 1 tablespoon smoked paprika

• ½ teaspoon salt, divided, plus a pinch

• 1 (15 ounce) can no-salt-added chickpeas, rinsed

• ⅓ cup buttermilk

• ¼ cup mayonnaise

• ¼ cup chopped fresh chives and/or dill, plus more for garnish

• ½ teaspoon ground pepper, divided

• ¼ teaspoon garlic powder

• 10 cups chopped kale

• ¼ cup water

• 1 ¼ pounds wild salmon, cut into 4 portions

Instructions:

1. Position racks in upper third and middle of oven; preheat to 425 degrees F.

2. Combine 1 tablespoon oil, paprika and 1/4 teaspoon salt in a medium bowl. Very thoroughly pat chickpeas dry, then toss with the paprika mixture. Spread on a rimmed baking sheet. Bake the chickpeas on the upper rack, stirring twice, for 30 minutes.

3. Meanwhile, puree buttermilk, mayonnaise, herbs, 1/4 teaspoon pepper and garlic powder in a blender until smooth. Set aside.

4. Heat the remaining 1 tablespoon oil in a large skillet over medium heat. Add kale and cook, stirring occasionally, for 2 minutes. Add water and continue cooking until the kale is tender, about 5 minutes more. Remove from heat and stir in a pinch of salt.

5. Remove the chickpeas from the oven and push them to one side of the pan. Place salmon on the other side and season with the remaining 1/4 teaspoon each salt and pepper. Bake until the salmon is just cooked through, 5 to 8 minutes.

6. Drizzle the reserved dressing on the salmon, garnish with more herbs, if desired, and serve with the kale and chickpeas.

Sheet-Pan Chili-Lime Salmon with Potatoes and Peppers

Ingredients:

• 1 pound Yukon Gold potatoes, cut into 3/4-inch pieces

• 2 tablespoons extra-virgin olive oil, divided

• ¾ teaspoon salt, divided

• ¼ teaspoon ground pepper

• 2 teaspoons chili powder

• 1 teaspoon ground cumin

• ½ teaspoon garlic powder

• 1 lime, zested and quartered

• 2 medium bell peppers, any color, sliced

• 1 ¼ pounds center-cut salmon fillet, skinned, if desired, and cut into 4 portions

Instructions:

1. Preheat oven to 425 degrees F. Coat a large rimmed baking sheet with cooking spray.

2. Toss potatoes, 1 tablespoon oil, 1/4 teaspoon salt and pepper together in a medium bowl. Transfer to the prepared pan and roast for 15 minutes.

3. Meanwhile, combine chili powder, cumin, garlic powder, lime zest and the remaining 1/2 teaspoon salt in a small bowl. Place bell peppers in the medium bowl and add the remaining 1 tablespoon oil and 1/2 tablespoon of the spice mixture; toss well to coat. Coat the salmon with the remaining spice mixture.

4. After 15 minutes, remove the pan from the oven. Add the peppers and stir to combine. Roast for 5 minutes. Remove from the oven; move some of the vegetables over and add the salmon to the pan. Roast until the salmon is just cooked through, 6 to 8 minutes. Serve with lime wedges.

Peppery Barbecue-Glazed Shrimp with Vegetables and Orzo

Ingredients:

• 1 pound peeled and deveined jumbo shrimp, thawed if frozen

• 1 teaspoon paprika

• ½ teaspoon garlic powder

- ½ teaspoon dried oregano, crushed

- ¼ teaspoon ground pepper

- ⅛ teaspoon cayenne pepper

- 1 cup whole-grain orzo

- 3 scallions

- 2 tablespoons olive oil, divided

- 2 cups coarsely chopped zucchini

- 1 cup coarsely chopped bell pepper

- ½ cup thinly sliced celery

- 1 cup cherry tomatoes, halved

- ½ teaspoon salt

- 2 tablespoons barbecue sauce

- Lemon wedges for serving

Instructions:

1. Place shrimp in a medium bowl. Combine paprika, garlic powder, oregano, pepper and cayenne in a small bowl. Sprinkle the spice mixture over the shrimp; toss to coat and set aside.

2. Bring a large saucepan of water to a boil. Cook orzo according to package directions; drain. Return to the hot pot; cover and keep warm.

3. Meanwhile, slice scallions, separating white and green parts. Heat 1 tablespoon oil in a medium skillet over medium-high heat. Add the scallion whites, zucchini, bell pepper and celery; cook, stirring occasionally, until the vegetables are crisp-tender, about 5 minutes. Add tomatoes; cook until softened, 2 to 3 minutes more. Add the vegetables to the pot with the orzo. Add salt; toss to combine.

4. In same skillet, heat the remaining 1 tablespoon oil over medium heat. Add the shrimp; cook, turning once, until opaque, 4 to 6 minutes. Drizzle with barbecue sauce. Cook and stir until the shrimp are coated, about 1 minute.

5. Serve the shrimp with the vegetable mixture. Top with scallion greens and serve with lemon wedges, if desired.

Chickpea Pasta with Mushrooms and Kale

Ingredients:

- 8 ounces chickpea rotini or penne

- ¼ cup extra-virgin olive oil

- 2 large cloves garlic, sliced

- Pinch of crushed red pepper

- 8 cups chopped kale

- 8 ounces cremini mushrooms, quartered

- ½ teaspoon dried thyme

- ½ teaspoon salt

- Grated Parmesan cheese for serving (optional)

Instructions:

1. Cook pasta according to package directions. Reserve 1 cup of the cooking water, then drain.

2. Meanwhile, heat oil in a large skillet over medium heat. Add garlic and crushed red pepper; cook, stirring once, until fragrant, about 1 minute. Add kale, mushrooms, thyme and salt; cook, stirring occasionally, until the vegetables are soft, about 5 minutes.

3. Stir in the pasta and enough of the reserved water to coat; cook, stirring, until combined and hot, about 1 minute more. Serve topped with Parmesan, if desired.

Ingredients:

- 14 large cloves garlic, divided

- ¼ cup extra-virgin olive oil

- 2 tablespoons finely chopped fresh oregano, divided

- 1 teaspoon salt, divided

- ¾ teaspoon freshly ground pepper, divided

- 6 cups Brussels sprouts, trimmed and sliced

- ¾ cup white wine, preferably Chardonnay

- 2 pounds wild-caught salmon fillet, skinned, cut into 6 portions

- Lemon wedges

Instructions:

1. Preheat oven to 450 degrees F.

2. Mince 2 garlic cloves and combine in a small bowl with oil, 1 tablespoon oregano, 1/2 teaspoon salt and 1/4 teaspoon pepper.

3. Halve the remaining garlic and toss with Brussels sprouts and 3 tablespoons of the seasoned oil in a large roasting pan. Roast, stirring once, for 15 minutes.

4. Add wine to the remaining oil mixture. Remove the pan from oven, stir the vegetables and place salmon on top. Drizzle with the wine mixture. Sprinkle with the remaining 1 tablespoon oregano and 1/2 teaspoon each salt and pepper.

5. Bake until the salmon is just cooked through, 5 to 10 minutes more. Serve with lemon wedges.

Berry Yogurt Parfait

Ingredients:

• 1 cup non-fat Greek yogurt

• 1/2 cup mixed berries (strawberries, blueberries, raspberries)

• 2 tablespoons granola

• 1 tablespoon honey or maple syrup (optional)

Instructions:

1. In a glass or bowl, layer Greek yogurt, mixed berries, and granola.

2. Drizzle with honey or maple syrup for added sweetness if desired. Repeat the layering if preferred and serve chilled.

Dark Chocolate-Dipped Strawberries

Ingredients:

• 1 cup fresh strawberries, rinsed and dried

• 2 oz dark chocolate (70% cocoa or higher)

Instructions:

1. Line a baking sheet with parchment paper.

2. In a microwave-safe bowl, melt the dark chocolate in 30-second intervals, stirring until smooth.

3. Hold each strawberry by the stem and dip it into the melted chocolate, coating about three-quarters of the strawberry.

4. Place the chocolate-dipped strawberries on the prepared baking sheet.

5. Let them set in the refrigerator for about 20-30 minutes before serving.

Frozen Banana Bites

Ingredients:

• 2 ripe bananas

• 1/4 cup unsweetened peanut butter or almond butter

• 1/4 cup shredded coconut or chopped nuts (optional)

• Popsicle sticks or toothpicks

Instructions:

1. Peel the bananas and cut them into bite-sized pieces.

2. Spread peanut butter or almond butter on one side of each banana piece.

3. If using, roll the peanut butter-coated banana pieces in shredded coconut or chopped nuts. Place a popsicle stick or toothpick into each banana bite.

4. Arrange the banana bites on a parchment-lined tray and freeze for at least 2 hours before serving.

Baked Cinnamon Apple Slices

Ingredients:

• 2 apples, cored and thinly sliced

• 1 tablespoon melted coconut oil or unsalted butter

• 1 teaspoon ground cinnamon

• 1 tablespoon honey or maple syrup (optional)

Instructions:

1. Preheat the oven to 350°F (175°C).

2. Toss the apple slices in melted coconut oil or unsalted butter.

3. Arrange the apple slices in a single layer on a baking sheet lined with parchment paper.

4. Sprinkle ground cinnamon over the apple slices. Drizzle with honey or maple syrup for added sweetness if desired.

5. Bake for 20-25 minutes or until the apples are tender and slightly caramelized. Let them cool for a few minutes before serving.

Mixed Berry Frozen Yogurt Bark

Ingredients:

• 2 cups non-fat Greek yogurt

• 1 cup mixed berries (strawberries, blueberries, raspberries)

• 2 tablespoons honey or maple syrup

• 2 tablespoons unsweetened shredded coconut (optional)

Instructions:

1. Line a baking sheet with parchment paper.

2. In a bowl, mix Greek yogurt and honey or maple syrup until well combined.

3. Spread the yogurt mixture evenly onto the prepared baking sheet.

4. Sprinkle mixed berries and shredded coconut over the yogurt. Freeze for 3-4 hours or until firm.

5. Break the frozen yogurt bark into pieces and serve immediately.

Banana-Oatmeal Cookies

Ingredients:

• 2 ripe bananas, mashed

• 1 cup rolled oats

• 1/4 cup unsweetened applesauce

• 1/4 cup chopped nuts (walnuts, almonds)

• 1/4 cup raisins or dried cranberries

• 1 teaspoon vanilla extract

• 1 teaspoon ground cinnamon

Instructions:

1. Preheat the oven to 350°F (175°C). Line a baking sheet with parchment paper.

2. In a bowl, combine mashed bananas, rolled oats, unsweetened applesauce, chopped nuts, raisins or dried cranberries, vanilla extract, and ground cinnamon.

3. Drop spoonfuls of the mixture onto the prepared baking sheet. Flatten the cookies slightly with a fork.

4. Bake for 15-20 minutes or until the cookies are golden brown.

5. Let them cool before serving.

Chia Seed Pudding with Berries

Ingredients:

• 1/4 cup chia seeds

• 1 cup unsweetened almond milk

• 1 tablespoon honey or maple syrup

• 1/2 teaspoon vanilla extract

• 1/2 cup mixed berries (strawberries, blueberries, raspberries)

Instructions:

1. In a bowl, mix chia seeds, unsweetened almond milk, honey or maple syrup, and vanilla extract.

2. Whisk well to combine and prevent clumping.

3. Let the mixture sit for 5 minutes, then whisk again to break up any clumps.

4. Cover and refrigerate for at least 2 hours or overnight until the mixture thickens into a pudding-like consistency.

5. Serve the chia seed pudding topped with mixed berries.

Apple Cinnamon Baked Oatmeal Cups

Ingredients:

• 2 cups rolled oats

• 1 teaspoon baking powder

• 1 teaspoon ground cinnamon

• 1/4 teaspoon salt

• 2 ripe bananas, mashed

• 1 cup unsweetened applesauce

- 1/2 cup unsweetened almond milk

- 1 apple, diced

- 2 tablespoons chopped nuts (optional)

Instructions:

1. Preheat the oven to 350°F (175°C). Grease a muffin tin.

2. In a bowl, mix rolled oats, baking powder, ground cinnamon, and salt.

3. Add mashed bananas, unsweetened applesauce, unsweetened almond milk, diced apple, and chopped nuts (if using). Stir until combined.

4. Spoon the mixture into the prepared muffin tin, filling each cup.

5. Bake for 25-30 minutes or until the oatmeal cups are set and golden brown.

6. Allow them to cool in the muffin tin for a few minutes before removing. Serve warm or at room temperature.

Greek Yogurt Berry Popsicles

Ingredients:

- 1 cup non-fat Greek yogurt

- 1 cup mixed berries (strawberries, blueberries, raspberries)

- 2 tablespoons honey or maple syrup

- Popsicle molds or small paper cups

- Popsicle sticks

Instructions:

1. In a blender, combine Greek yogurt, mixed berries, and honey or maple syrup. Blend until smooth.

2. Pour the mixture into popsicle molds or small paper cups.

3. Place a popsicle stick in the center of each mold. Freeze for at least 4-6 hours until the popsicles are firm.

4. Run the molds under warm water for a few seconds to release the popsicles before serving.

Mango Sorbet

Ingredients:

- 2 ripe mangoes, peeled and diced

- 1 tablespoon honey or maple syrup

• 2 tablespoons fresh lime juice

• 1/4 cup water

Instructions:

1. Place diced mangoes, honey or maple syrup, fresh lime juice, and water in a blender or food processor.

2. Blend until smooth and creamy.

3. Pour the mixture into a shallow dish or container and cover with plastic wrap.

4. Freeze for at least 3-4 hours, stirring every hour to break up ice crystals and maintain a smooth texture.

5. Serve the mango sorbet scooped into bowls.

Almond Butter Banana Bites

Ingredients:

• 2 ripe bananas, sliced

• 1/4 cup almond butter

• 2 tablespoons unsweetened shredded coconut

• 2 tablespoons chopped almonds (optional)

Instructions:

1. Spread almond butter on banana slices.

2. Sprinkle shredded coconut and chopped almonds (if using) over the almond butter.

3. Place a toothpick in each banana slice. Serve immediately or freeze for a firmer texture.

Greek Yogurt Fruit Dip

Ingredients:

• 1 cup non-fat Greek yogurt

• 1 tablespoon honey or maple syrup

• 1/2 teaspoon vanilla extract

• Assorted fruit for dipping (strawberries, apple slices, pineapple chunks)

Instructions:

1. In a bowl, mix Greek yogurt, honey or maple syrup, and vanilla extract until well combined.

2. Serve the Greek yogurt dip alongside the assorted fruit for dipping.

Baked Apples with Cinnamon and Walnuts

Ingredients:

• 2 apples, cored and halved

• 2 tablespoons chopped walnuts

• 1 tablespoon honey or maple syrup

• 1/2 teaspoon ground cinnamon

Instructions:

1. Preheat the oven to 375°F (190°C).

2. Place apple halves on a baking sheet lined with parchment paper.

3. In a small bowl, mix chopped walnuts, honey or maple syrup, and ground cinnamon. Fill the core of each apple half with the walnut mixture.

4. Bake for 20-25 minutes or until the apples are tender.

5. Serve the baked apples warm.

Berry Frozen Yogurt Bites

Ingredients:

• 1 cup non-fat Greek yogurt

• 1/2 cup mixed berries (strawberries, blueberries, raspberries)

• 1 tablespoon honey or maple syrup

Instructions:

1. In a bowl, mix Greek yogurt and honey or maple syrup until smooth. Gently fold in the mixed berries.

2. Spoon small dollops of the yogurt mixture onto a baking sheet lined with parchment paper.

3. Freeze for 2-3 hours or until the yogurt bites are firm. Serve the frozen yogurt bites chilled.

Chocolate Avocado Pudding

Ingredients:

• 2 ripe avocados, peeled and pitted

• 1/4 cup unsweetened cocoa powder

• 1/4 cup honey or maple syrup

• 1 teaspoon vanilla extract

Instructions:

1. In a blender or food processor, blend avocados, cocoa powder, honey or maple syrup, and vanilla extract until smooth and creamy.

2. Spoon the chocolate avocado pudding into serving bowls.

3. Refrigerate for at least 30 minutes before serving.

Mixed Berry Frozen Yogurt

Ingredients:

• 2 cups plain non-fat Greek yogurt

• 2 cups mixed berries (strawberries, blueberries, raspberries)

• 1-2 tablespoons honey or maple syrup (optional)

Instructions:

1. In a blender, combine Greek yogurt, mixed berries, and honey or maple syrup (if desired).

2. Blend until smooth. Pour the mixture into a freezer-safe container.

3. Freeze for 4-6 hours or until firm. Allow it to soften for a few minutes before serving.

Peanut Butter Banana Ice Cream

Ingredients:

- 4 ripe bananas, sliced and frozen

- 2 tablespoons peanut butter (unsweetened)

- 1-2 tablespoons unsweetened cocoa powder (optional)

Instructions:

1. Place the frozen banana slices in a food processor.

2. Add peanut butter (and cocoa powder if desired).

3. Pulse until the mixture is smooth and creamy, scraping down the sides as needed.

4. Serve immediately for a soft-serve texture or freeze for 30 minutes for a firmer consistency.

Coconut Chia Seed Pudding

Ingredients:

- 1/4 cup chia seeds

- 1 cup unsweetened coconut milk

- 1 tablespoon honey or maple syrup

- 1/4 teaspoon vanilla extract

- Unsweetened shredded coconut and fresh berries for topping

Instructions:

1. In a bowl, mix chia seeds, coconut milk, honey or maple syrup, and vanilla extract.

2. Whisk well to combine and avoid clumps.

3. Refrigerate for at least 2 hours or until the mixture thickens into a pudding-like consistency.

4. Serve the chia seed pudding topped with shredded coconut and fresh berries.

Mango Coconut Sorbet

Ingredients:

- 2 ripe mangoes, peeled and diced

- 1 can (13.5 oz) unsweetened coconut milk

• 2 tablespoons honey or maple syrup

Instructions:

1. Place diced mangoes, unsweetened coconut milk, and honey or maple syrup in a blender. Blend until smooth.

2. Pour the mixture into a shallow dish or container and cover with plastic wrap.

3. Freeze for at least 4-6 hours, stirring occasionally for a smooth texture.

4. Serve scoops of mango coconut sorbet.

Frozen Berry Pops

Ingredients:

• 2 cups mixed berries (strawberries, blueberries, raspberries)

• 1 cup plain non-fat Greek yogurt

• 2 tablespoons honey or maple syrup

• Popsicle molds or small paper cups

• Popsicle sticks

Instructions:

1. In a blender, combine mixed berries, Greek yogurt, and honey or maple syrup. Blend until smooth.

2. Pour the mixture into popsicle molds or small paper cups.

3. Place a popsicle stick in the center of each mold. Freeze for at least 4 hours or until the popsicles are firm.

4. Run the molds under warm water for a few seconds to release the popsicles before serving.

Lemon Blueberry Chia Seed Pudding

Ingredients:

• 1/4 cup chia seeds

• 1 cup unsweetened almond milk

• Zest and juice of 1 lemon

• 1 tablespoon honey or maple syrup

• 1/2 cup fresh blueberries

Instructions:

1. In a bowl, mix chia seeds, almond milk, lemon zest, lemon juice, and honey or maple syrup.

2. Whisk well and let it sit for 5 minutes, then whisk again to avoid clumping.

3. Refrigerate for at least 2 hours or overnight until the mixture thickens into a pudding-like consistency.

4. Before serving, layer the chia seed pudding and fresh blueberries in serving glasses or bowls.

Apple Cinnamon Quinoa Bites

Ingredients:

• 1 cup cooked quinoa

• 1 apple, finely diced

• 1/4 cup unsweetened applesauce

• 1 teaspoon ground cinnamon

• 1 tablespoon honey or maple syrup

• 1/4 cup chopped walnuts or almonds

Instructions:

1. Preheat the oven to 350°F (175°C). Grease a mini-muffin tin.

2. In a bowl, mix cooked quinoa, diced apple, unsweetened applesauce, ground cinnamon, honey or maple syrup, and chopped nuts.

3. Spoon the mixture into the mini-muffin tin, filling each cup.

4. Bake for 20-25 minutes or until golden brown.

5. Allow them to cool in the muffin tin for a few minutes before removing. Serve warm or at room temperature.

Peach and Berry Crisp

Ingredients:

- 4 cups sliced peaches

- 1 cup mixed berries (strawberries, blueberries)

- 1 tablespoon honey or maple syrup

- 1 teaspoon ground cinnamon

- 1/2 cup rolled oats

- 1/4 cup almond flour

- 2 tablespoons chopped almonds

- 2 tablespoons unsalted butter or coconut oil, melted

Instructions:

1. Preheat the oven to 375°F (190°C). Grease a baking dish.

2. In a bowl, toss sliced peaches and mixed berries with honey or maple syrup and ground cinnamon.

3. Spread the fruit mixture evenly in the prepared baking dish.

4. In another bowl, combine rolled oats, almond flour, chopped almonds, and melted butter or coconut oil. Sprinkle the oat mixture over the fruit.

5. Bake for 25-30 minutes or until the topping is golden brown and the fruit is bubbling.

6. Let it cool slightly before serving.

Pineapple Coconut Nice Cream

Ingredients:

- 2 cups frozen pineapple chunks

- 1 can (13.5 oz) unsweetened coconut milk

- 2 tablespoons honey or maple syrup

- 1/4 cup shredded coconut (optional)

Instructions:

1. In a blender, blend frozen pineapple chunks, coconut milk, and honey or maple syrup until smooth.

2. Add shredded coconut (if using) and pulse a few times to mix.

3. Serve the pineapple coconut nice cream immediately for a soft-serve texture or freeze for 30 minutes for a firmer consistency.

4. Garnish with additional shredded coconut before serving if desired.

Chocolate-Dipped Banana Pops

Ingredients:

• 2 ripe bananas, peeled and cut in half crosswise

• 4 oz dark chocolate (70% cocoa or higher), chopped

• 2 tablespoons chopped nuts (almonds, walnuts)

• Popsicle sticks

Instructions:

1. Insert a popsicle stick into each banana half.

2. Place the bananas on a parchment-lined baking sheet and freeze for 1-2 hours until firm.

3. Melt the dark chocolate in a microwave-safe bowl in 30-second intervals, stirring until smooth.

4. Dip each frozen banana half into the melted chocolate, then sprinkle with chopped nuts.

5. Place the chocolate-dipped banana pops back on the baking sheet and freeze until the chocolate is set.

6. Serve the banana pops chilled.

Strawberry Yogurt Bark

Ingredients:

- 2 cups plain non-fat Greek yogurt

- 1 cup fresh strawberries, sliced

- 2 tablespoons honey or maple syrup

- 2 tablespoons unsweetened shredded coconut (optional)

Instructions:

1. Line a baking sheet with parchment paper.

2. In a bowl, mix Greek yogurt and honey or maple syrup until smooth. Spread the yogurt mixture evenly onto the prepared baking sheet.

3. Arrange sliced strawberries on top of the yogurt. Sprinkle unsweetened shredded coconut (if using) over the strawberries.

4. Freeze for 3-4 hours or until firm. Break the frozen yogurt bark into pieces before serving.

Mango Lime Sorbet

Ingredients:

• 2 ripe mangoes, peeled and diced

• Juice of 2 limes

• 2 tablespoons honey or maple syrup

• 1/4 cup water

Instructions:

1. Place diced mangoes, lime juice, honey or maple syrup, and water in a blender. Blend until smooth.

2. Pour the mixture into a shallow dish or container and cover with plastic wrap.

3. Freeze for at least 4-6 hours, stirring occasionally for a smooth texture.

4. Serve scoops of mango lime sorbet.

Almond Date Energy Bites

Ingredients:

- 1 cup pitted dates

- 1 cup rolled oats

- 1/4 cup almond butter (unsweetened)

- 1/4 cup chopped almonds

- 1 tablespoon chia seeds

- 1 teaspoon vanilla extract

- Unsweetened shredded coconut for coating (optional)

Instructions:

1. In a food processor, blend dates until they form a paste-like consistency.

2. Add rolled oats, almond butter, chopped almonds, chia seeds, and vanilla extract. Pulse until well combined.

3. Roll the mixture into small bite-sized balls.

4. Optional: Roll the energy bites in unsweetened shredded coconut to coat.

5. Refrigerate for at least 30 minutes before serving.

Blueberry Lemon Frozen Yogurt

Ingredients:

• 2 cups plain non-fat Greek yogurt

• 1 cup fresh or frozen blueberries

• Zest and juice of 1 lemon

• 2-3 tablespoons honey or maple syrup

Instructions:

1. In a blender, combine Greek yogurt, blueberries, lemon zest, lemon juice, and honey or maple syrup.

2. Blend until smooth. Pour the mixture into a freezer-safe container.

3. Freeze for 4-6 hours or until firm. Allow it to soften for a few minutes before serving.

Banana Walnut "Ice Cream"

Ingredients:

- 4 ripe bananas, sliced and frozen

- 1/4 cup chopped walnuts

- 1 tablespoon honey or maple syrup

Instructions:

1. Place the frozen banana slices in a food processor. Add chopped walnuts and honey or maple syrup.

2. Pulse until the mixture is creamy and resembles ice cream.

3. Serve immediately for a soft-serve texture or freeze for 30 minutes for a firmer consistency.

CONCLUSION

In conclusion, exploring the Dietary Approaches to Stop Hypertension (DASH) diet unveils a versatile and balanced approach to healthy eating. The comprehensive guidelines and principles outlined within this dietary regimen underscore its efficacy not only in managing blood pressure but also as a well-rounded strategy for weight management and overall health improvement.

The DASH diet emphasizes the consumption of nutrient-dense foods, such as fruits, vegetables, whole grains, lean proteins, and low-fat dairy, while limiting sodium, saturated fats, and added sugars. Its foundation lies in promoting heart health, reducing the risk of chronic diseases, and fostering sustainable weight loss.

Additionally, integrating physical activity alongside this dietary approach is paramount for maximizing its benefits. The combination of healthy eating and regular exercise serves as a robust strategy for achieving and maintaining overall wellness.

From breakfast, lunch to dinner and dessert options, the provided recipes exemplify the creativity and variety attainable within the DASH diet framework. These nutrient-packed recipes underscore the delightful possibilities while adhering to the diet's principles, enabling individuals to indulge in flavorful yet health-conscious meals and desserts.

Embracing the DASH diet is not merely a short-term endeavor but a sustainable lifestyle choice. Overcoming challenges, staying motivated, and fostering accountability are pivotal elements in successfully adhering to this dietary regimen.

In essence, the DASH diet transcends a mere weight loss solution. It stands as a holistic approach to well-being, fostering healthier habits that can positively impact one's life. By emphasizing wholesome, delicious, and nutritious foods, coupled with an active lifestyle, the DASH diet paves the way for individuals to achieve improved health and vitality in the long run.

9 798872 347231